**NO LONGER PROPERTY OF
SEATTLE PUBLIC LIBRARY** RECEIVED

APR 2 0 2018

BROADVIEW LIBRARY

PRAISE FOR *YOGA & PSYCHE*

"As we gain greater understanding about the body's response to psychological wounding, the integration of psychotherapy with body-based introspective wisdom traditions is producing new, more effective pathways to healing from trauma. This book is an important contribution to that endeavor. It is clearly written and comprehensively researched, providing a valuable resource of information and insight."

JUDITH BLACKSTONE, PHD
founder of the Realization Process and author
of *Belonging Here* and *The Intimate Life*

"Seamlessly weaving yoga, neuroscience, somatics, and psychotherapy with the latest research, Mariana's work is ~~accessible~~ and intelligent. She integrates yoga a~~~~ ~~~~ries and hands-on practices to generate~~~~ ~~~~on."

~~~~ER

a~~~~ *You*

"Mariana Caplan is a highly integrative thinker and writer, and in her new book, *Yoga & Psyche*, she has given us an extremely useful, detailed, and much-needed look at the current interface between the worlds of psychotherapy and yoga. These two worlds—and their oft-differing views about the nature of human possibility—have been interacting much more frequently over the past several decades, but not always with clarity. Dr. Caplan brings this much-needed clarity in her very comprehensive new book. She skillfully examines the latest breakthroughs in neuroscience, trauma theory, and physiology in ways that shed tremendous light on the real challenges that face the contemporary practitioner of yoga, meditation, and the contemplative arts. All of us in the field should be most grateful for this book, which will certainly become a must-read in the field."

STEPHEN COPE
Senior Scholar-in-Residence at Kripalu Center for Yoga and Health, and
author of *Yoga and the Quest for the True Self* and *The Wisdom of Yoga*

NO LONGER PROPERTY OF
SEATTLE PUBLIC LIBRARY

"In this clear, comprehensive, and touchingly personal guide, Mariana Caplan unites ancient and contemporary maps to the journey into full humanity. Through rigorous research and unflinching personal inquiry, she has created an indispensable resource for yoga teachers and students, psychotherapists and clients, and any spiritual seeker who wants to illuminate the shadows of their chosen path."

ANNE CUSHMAN
author of *Enlightenment for Idiots: A Novel* and *Moving into Meditation*

"To claim our genuine inheritance as fully integrated human beings, capable of navigating the intricacies of everyday life, we must achieve both spiritual and psychological competency. Unfortunately, the two paths of spiritual awakening and psychological integration have often been viewed as separate undertakings. Too often yoga has emphasized spiritual competency while neglecting psychological integration, and psychological exploration has left spiritual self-realization by the wayside. *Yoga & Psyche* strikes a resonate chord for our modern era by recognizing the necessity of embracing both psychological and spiritual realization in order for us to embody our true potential as fully awake human beings. Caplan offers us a comprehensive view that includes both path and means for attaining true spiritual realization and in-depth psychological integration that respects all aspects of our body, mind, cognitions, emotions, and spirit. *Yoga & Psyche* shows us how to truly embrace and embody our true potential as fully awake and alive human beings."

RICHARD MILLER, PHD
author of *iRest Meditation: Restorative Practices
for Health, Resiliency, and Well-Being*

YOGA & PSYCHE

INTEGRATING THE PATHS OF YOGA AND PSYCHOLOGY FOR HEALING, TRANSFORMATION, AND JOY

MARIANA CAPLAN, PhD, MFT

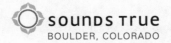

BOULDER, COLORADO

Sounds True
Boulder, CO 80306

© 2018 Mariana Caplan
Chapter 5 © 2018 by Mariana Caplan and Gabriel Axel
Foreword © 2018 Don Hanlon Johnson

Sounds True is a trademark of Sounds True, Inc. All rights reserved. No part of this book may be used or reproduced in any manner without written permission from the author(s) and publisher.

Published 2018

This book is not intended as a substitute for the medical recommendations of physicians, mental-health professionals, or other health-care providers. Rather, it is intended to offer information to help the reader cooperate with physicians, mental-health professionals, and health-care providers in a mutual quest for optimal well-being. We advise readers to carefully review and understand the ideas presented and to seek the advice of a qualified professional before attempting to use them.

Some names and identifying details have been changed to protect the privacy of individuals.

Cover design by Jennifer Miles
Book design by Beth Skelley

Printed in Canada

Library of Congress Cataloging-in-Publication Data
Names: Caplan, Mariana, 1969- author.
Title: Yoga & psyche : integrating the paths of yoga and psychology
   for healing, transformation, and joy / Mariana Caplan, PhD, MFT.
Other titles: Yoga and psyche
Description: Boulder, CO : Sounds True, Inc., [2018] | Includes
   bibliographical references.
Identifiers: LCCN 2017024882 (print) | LCCN 2017049459 (ebook) |
   ISBN 9781622037261 (ebook) | ISBN 9781622036561 (pbk.)
Subjects: LCSH: Psychology. | Yoga. | Mental healing.
Classification: LCC BF121 (ebook) | LCC BF121 .C337 2018 (print) |
   DDC 613.7/046—dc23
LC record available at https://lccn.loc.gov/2017024882

10 9 8 7 6 5 4 3 2 1

For Zion ~ my Promised Land

In loving memory of Georg Feuerstein (1947–2012) ~
a great scholar of yoga, mentor, and heart friend

CONTENTS

FOREWORD

by Don Hanlon Johnson, PhD

While reading this manuscript, I thought of Yo-Yo Ma's inaugural speech for the opening of his Silk Road Project at the turn of the century. He had discovered that musicians all along the Silk Road from Kamchatka to Prague value playing with one another, despite their strangeness to one another, because over centuries they have learned that meeting others with different instruments, lyrics, tonalities, and melodies is a source of constantly renewing inspiration. While Muslims, Christians, Marxists, and other politically minded communities along the great road continue to engage in slaughter and persecution, it is the musicians, singers, and dancers who know how to work together to create moments of great beauty.

Something similar has been occurring recently in the West in a field I am more familiar with: somatics, particularly embodiment practices. Teachers and practitioners of all types of dance, massage, Capoeira, Qi Gong, Authentic Movement, Rolfing, Candomblé, and countless other paths have come together to find new inspiration. Here too, we see people from widely different backgrounds—even from ordinarily contentious groups—opening up to each other, sharing their expertise, and co-creating new experiences of movement, breathing, and sound.

At the same time, it takes a Mariana Caplan and others like her to bring to fruition what is only now beginning to emerge as a global community of practice. I've had the pleasure of being long-term colleagues with Mariana at the California Institute of Integral Studies, where I founded the somatics program in 1983 after working with Ida Rolf and visionaries in the fields of Feldenkrais, sensory awareness,

Orgonomy, Middendorf Breath Work, Continuum Movement, body-mind centering, osteopathy, and many others to create a new approach to healing the mind-body split that continues to plague today's world. As this book will make clear, Mariana has long been committed to similar work, albeit as a pioneer in articulating the profound implications of the union between psychology and spiritual practice—specifically yoga.

Yo-Yo Ma could have remained successful within the highly refined yet tightly bound communities devoted to Vivaldi, Bach, and Mozart. But he dared to venture out of that brilliant and well-funded world into the broader worlds of Tajikistan, China, and the Caucasus, constantly finding new instrumentalists to engage with and bring with him to play around the world. Similarly, Mariana could have blossomed in either field of her expertise, but she chose to explore, encourage, and integrate the links between yoga and psychology.

Among gifted teachers, there is a tendency to insist on the correctness of their particular *way*. What's missing in this tethered approach, however, is the creation of something greater than one's personal vision or tradition will allow. With the offering of *Yoga & Psyche*, Mariana invites us to share in the joys of collaborative investigation in order to birth a new field in which experts in psychology, somatics, yoga, trauma research, and neuroscience all have a place.

It's significant to note that Mariana is not merely an academic, but a dedicated, lifelong practitioner and student of the traditions she explores here. Her writing conveys a particular intimacy, and simultaneously transmits that rare spaciousness of someone who appreciates the amazing diversity of human ingenuities. She and her team have been engaged in research that traverses international borders and fields of study in order to connect individuals and groups who share a focus on embodied approaches to crafting a more satisfying life and healing from the ravages of personal and collective trauma. And this particular book is unique in that it is perhaps the most thorough of its kind to present the integration of yoga and psychology from academic, clinical, and personal perspectives. Finally, in fields typically associated with pioneering men from Vienna and India, Mariana offers an uncommon and too-often ignored viewpoint as a woman. Doing so, she claims her place among the growing community of leaders dedicated to crafting a global, embodied psychology.

Yoga has reached the point where it has thoroughly permeated our culture. Here in the United States, it seems that even small towns have at least one yoga studio, and practicing yoga asanas is now widely considered to be complementary of other spiritual traditions in a way that would have been unthinkable mere decades ago. Furthermore, yoga has become quite popular among celebrities, professional athletes, and entrepreneurs. Sadly, the profound riches of yoga can easily be missed, as it is marketed as yet another commodity to make one thinner, more attractive, peaceful, and so on.

In a similar way, psychology has saturated the values and vocabulary of the West, and therapy—once associated primarily with severe mental distress—is commonly engaged by people of all economic, political, and religious backgrounds. Yet here too, the promise of psychology can easily be reduced to self-improvement.

Even among the most dedicated of followers, neither yoga nor psychology alone offers a complete approach to integrated psychological and spiritual transformation. As Mariana explains, yoga by itself "does not heal relational wounds, increase self-esteem, enhance communication, reveal or change self-destructive patterns, or end addictions." While Western psychology does address these problems, by itself psychology "can't offer the contentment, joy, and life-altering experiences that yoga and other spiritual practices can." It's easy to see how either path alone can lack something crucial, and how both—when integrated—can generate something remarkable, fresh, and uncommonly beneficial.

For this reason, *Yoga & Psyche* is generative and groundbreaking. Mariana not only illustrates the obvious worth of following each path in an integrated way, she also elucidates how yoga and psychology can be informed by the related fields of somatics, neuroscience, and trauma studies, and she does so with an accessible voice that offers hands-on practices. Finally, Mariana provides a vision of how those of us working from different standpoints can engage more fruitfully with each other in shaping a more humane world in such a dangerous and delicate time in human history.

INTRODUCTION

Not knowing when the Dawn will come,
I open every Door[1]
EMILY DICKINSON

Yoga saved half my life; psychology saved the other. Yoga became my passion, vision, friend, lifeline, and half of my vocation. It also brought me tremendous depth, dimension, joy, and health on multiple levels. I'm not alone in this, of course: there are innumerable stories of yogis, teachers, and longtime practitioners who arrived at yoga through crises. Yoga restored them, rebalanced them, and gave them new inspiration and fulfillment.

And just as innumerable people credit yoga with saving their lives, the same is true of psychology. The growing evolution of psychology and psychotherapy—particularly with the advances in neuroscience, somatics, and trauma research—has brought countless lives from imbalance into balance, neurosis into well-being, and surviving into thriving. Through the myriad forms of counseling, psychiatry, and psychologically informed transformational processes, psychology has and will continue to help individuals work through anxiety, depression, addiction, issues in intimate relationships, parenting, interpersonal and existential challenges, and various other psychological realities that most of us face at some point or another in our lives. For me, psychology and yoga are lifelong friends that never let me down when the going gets rough.

When my child was only eighteen months old, I felt compelled to write this book, which meant synthesizing abundant research with what I personally had learned from two decades of work in psychology and yoga. I became eager to know who else in the world was working with these subjects and what would happen if we pooled our knowledge and insights cross-culturally, collaborating to share and integrate the best of each other's wisdom and discoveries. One of my early mentors, a pioneering sociologist and author named Joseph Chilton Pearce, once told me that whenever he truly wanted to learn about something, he would write a book about it. He said that the process of putting a book together meant access to new people all around the world, including their feedback and collective resources, which would eventually synthesize into another book, and this nourished Joe's commitment to lifelong learning. In a similar way, I want to connect with amazing people who love the same subjects I do in order to co-create a new field that synthesizes the traditions of contemporary psychology and yoga. It feels inevitable and utterly exciting that these paths to healing can begin to meet and inform each other.

As the single mother of a young child, I had limited time to complete the necessary research, so I reached out for help. I asked for one or two volunteer assistants to help amass all the academic research and popular writings done in these fields to date. To my surprise, more than twenty highly qualified applicants (mostly graduate students who studied and taught yoga) offered to help with the research. Since the assistance was so expert and abundant, we expanded the project to something greater than a single book, which is how the Yoga & Psyche Project was born. To date, this includes the publication of academic research, the first international Yoga & Psyche Conference (2014), the book *Proceedings from the Yoga & Psyche Conference (2014)*, a series of in-person and online workshops that people can participate in from anywhere in the world, and, most importantly, the beginnings of a global community coming together to co-create this new field of possibility for personal and planetary healing.

MY HEALING JOURNEY THROUGH YOGA AND PSYCHOLOGY

A large number of people come to my talks and workshops with an attraction to both psychology and yoga but with little sense of how the two might fit together. I am often stopped in my tracks when I remember this. I have been living so deeply with these two traditions for so long that I cannot remember a time when they were apart or different from each other. To me, they are so compatible that I often think of them as parents who have lovingly raised me, or like soul mates who are complete as individuals but who are so much happier together, or like best friends who always have each other's backs. At each turn in my life, when yoga opened up a new expansion, I turned to psychology to integrate a subsequent level of unconscious material. Likewise, when the next layer of psychological healing or opening revealed itself, yoga beckoned me to integrate it into its endless, expansive arms. For countless others and myself, this process of continual, mutual enhancement of psychological and yogic unfolding—symbolized by the lemniscate, or infinity sign—has never stopped. Each becomes greater through the inclusion of the other.

I stumbled onto the spiritual path as a nineteen-year-old. I was a wounded, passionate, and adventurous undergraduate student, hungry to make sense of my childhood and its pains, and eager to discover deeper meaning in life. During my first year at the University of Michigan, I learned that there was a whole "field" of spirituality beyond the ultra-conservative Judeo-Christian options presented to me as child. I jumped in with both feet first. I tried everything: Native American spirituality, shamanism, tai chi, Western philosophy, Hassidic Judaism, Buddhist meditation, Hindu devotional practices, African drumming, and a variety of New Age techniques. Sadly, I quickly experienced abundant contradictions and hypocrisy among the spiritual groups and teachers I encountered. The married, Native American sweat-lodge leader felt me up during a sacred ceremony while his beautiful wife and kids played outside. A particular shaman in Mexico attacked and nearly raped me. I lived for a summer in a van with an elder Christian mystic-activist and ended up replaying the worst of my childhood family dynamics and trauma.

By the time I was twenty-two, I had learned that the spiritual quest was deeply intertwined with unconscious psychological dynamics, and this realization led me to attend graduate school for counseling psychology. I chose a program that emphasized engaging in psychological inquiry, both within and outside the classroom. For three years, I pummeled my psyche in an effort to understand why I kept repeating childhood dynamics with boyfriends and spiritual teachers. I explored my intense emotions and nightmares, faced my existential fears of death, and sought to unravel the mysteries of my childhood traumas.

I remain passionate to this day about exploring the endless possibilities offered by what I call "depth psychology." (For me, what distinguishes depth psychology from many of the modern, mainstream, and short-therapy approaches to psychology is that both the therapist and client are committed to exploring the individual and his or her psyche at a deep level for a substantial period of time, often one to three years. Depth therapy also refers to a therapist's ongoing commitment to his or her own growth.)

When I finished grad school, however, I felt the pull to immerse myself in the study and practice of mystical traditions beyond psychology. Upon graduation, I purchased a one-way ticket to India in pursuit of the deepest spiritual longings of my heart and soul. Although I still lived with the pains caused by spiritual teachers in my early twenties, I still yearned to discover truly great gurus and mystics, explore intensive meditation and yoga practice, and delve into the sincere pursuit of God or Truth.

In India, alongside contradictions and hypocrisies in several teachers and seekers I came across, I was fortunate to meet Yogi Ramsuratkumar, the most extraordinary yogi I have ever encountered in my life. His blessings still influence me on a daily basis. I fully dedicated myself to a life of austere spiritual practice and community life for several years under Yogi Ramsuratkumar's guidance, and his American disciple, Lee Lozowick, became my spiritual teacher for sixteen years until Lee's death in 2010. Yogi Ramsuratkumar profoundly embodied what is possible through practicing inner yoga. He exemplified the spiritual life of someone on fire for Life, God, Truth, and Love, and he never ceased to burn and shine more as he aged, bringing profound compassion and awareness to thousands of people as he blazed ever further into the depths of consciousness and the cosmos. Among other things, Yogi Ramsuratkumar taught me that there is truly no end to the path. This lesson has protected me whenever I start to believe I have "arrived" somewhere on the spiritual path.

Although my spiritual teacher always insisted there was nothing wrong with me psychologically and that I did not *need* psychotherapy, I felt in my bones that I did. It was not enough for me to live a life of service at the ashram while still feeling trapped and miserable. It was not enough to repeat sabotaging patterns in intimate relationships while I continued to develop spiritually. And it was not enough to focus on ultimate spiritual truth while I still experienced strong symptoms of trauma of an unknown origin that cried out for attention. I needed yoga *and* psychology. Upon leaving the life of an ashram renunciant, I re-engaged with my doctoral and then postgraduate studies in psychology, somatics, and trauma as a client and as a professional, always in tandem with ongoing yogic studies. Ultimately, neither the psychological nor spiritual path alone offered what I needed to address the depths that felt necessary to unwind in order to experience the totality of my wholeness, my gifts, and my full capacity to love and be loved, to give and receive.

No amount of yoga, no particular spiritual tradition, no teacher or guru alone has been fully able to penetrate aspects of my own and others' psychological constitution in the way that psychotherapy and the important innovations in psychology have been able to. At the same time, deep psychological studies and inquiry do not by themselves take us to the depths, insights, connectedness, and embodied release that yoga and other profound mystical practices can. As I emphasize repeatedly in this book, these two remarkable traditions are not lacking in any way, but when they are practiced together they offer a greater spectrum of possibility than either of them alone—particularly for the Western individual.[2]

At the age of thirty-four, my body collapsed into a state of chronic fatigue, and I suffered from multiple autoimmune disorders, including a full-body pain that lasted for three years. My illness was compounded by periods of isolation, mental and physical impairment, and intermittent anxiety and depression. I feared I would never get better; or worse, that my health would decline even further. My pain was magnified by the terror of dying without having lived the possibilities of true love and motherhood. No matter what I did, I could not regain my health, and I lacked the energy to engage in any of my various passions.

For the first two years of my illness, I spent thousands of dollars visiting a variety of excellent physicians, both traditional and alternative, to varying degrees of improvement. Unfortunately, I always relapsed, and my disease was never accurately diagnosed. At some point, I decided it was necessary to discover my own "inner healer" (as New Agey as that sounded even to me at the time), understand my body at a whole new level, and learn to manage my healing process from within. In yoga, the deity Jangalikayamane represents the inner physician that yogis have accessed by practicing for long periods of time isolated in nature. I traveled to the Hawai'ian island of Kaua'i, intending to saturate myself in deep nature, water, and yoga in order to heal from within.

On Kaua'i, I immersed myself in hatha yoga and the healing environment of the island. I ate healthy and energizing foods, exercised, breathed, listened to my body, released tensions as they arose, and relaxed from the inside for what felt like the first time in my life. I had studied the esoteric aspects of yoga and meditation since meeting Yogi Ramsuratkumar over a decade before, but now a new door began to open through my body. I felt newly connected with the somatic—the deeply embodied—aspects of my experience, where my trauma and psychological conditioning intertwined with my physiology, posture, breath, and chronic body pains. In three short weeks, yoga enabled me to access deep wellsprings of healing, radiant energy, and life force that had lain latent in my body.

I sprang into health. And I saw and felt the profound and immediate effects of deeply listening to my body, learning to follow its directions, unwinding my illness from within. Aided by the healing waters and buoyantly fresh energy of the island, I enjoyed a remission that lasted throughout my trip; all of my symptoms almost fully disappeared. However, within days of my return to the mainland, my illness returned, escalating in intensity over the next several months. I was exhausted from three years of failed treatments. I couldn't eat, exercise, or work in any functional way. I felt desperate. I returned to Kaua'i in terrible condition, but entered a yoga teacher training that included intensive *asana* (posture), *pranayama* (breathing exercises), Sanskrit, philosophy, Ayurvedic fasts and cleanses, and Jyotish (yogic astrology). To support the effects of the yoga, I engaged in regular sessions of deep bodywork. My symptoms disappeared almost immediately, and my body began to strengthen rapidly.

I began to understand how much of my illness had been created by a deep imbalance in my life on many levels. Yoga means *balance* (among other things), and the more I balanced my life and energy, the healthier I became. My body went into a full and lasting remission, moving from sickness to vitality. I emerged stronger, more energetic and balanced, and happier than I had been before the illness began. Yoga healed my body and placed my life back on track. However, I knew that there were deep psychological layers of trauma and emotion still trapped in my body. Yoga had touched upon them, but it had not given me the tools to specifically address my Western psychological makeup.

At this time, I discovered somatic psychology and trauma healing, and I began and completed Peter Levine's Somatic Experiencing® training. Yoga landed me deep inside my body. It penetrated layers that were not only physical but spiritual. Even so, there were crevices of my psyche that were imprisoned within my body, and they had not been healed. They continued to express themselves by repeating negative life patterns that brought pain and unnecessary suffering to myself and others. Opening the doors of somatics in both my yoga and therapy practice was a major turning point in my life.

It has become increasingly clear to me and many of my contemporaries who are both psychologists and therapists—as well as dedicated teachers and students of yoga and other traditions—that spiritual practice and psychological inquiry simply do not replace each other. Spiritual practice can take people to heights of bliss, transcendence, oneness, emptiness, and mystical union in ways that nothing else can. However, by itself yoga does not heal relational wounds, increase self-esteem, enhance communication, reveal or change self-destructive patterns, or end addictions. Western psychology, on the other hand, does address these aspects of our shared humanity. Even so, psychology by itself can't offer the contentment, joy, and life-altering experiences that yoga and other spiritual practices can.

In 2006, I began to teach on the intersection of yoga and Western psychology. Since that time, I have developed the Yoga & Psyche Project, including multiple methods, a "toolbox," and various training programs. And I'm devoted to further research and continuing to refine the processes I offer as my experience matures and deepens. This book offers a culmination of my personal, professional, and spiritual inquiries into this profound and extraordinary new synthesis to date. It proposes that yoga and psychology create a deeper possibility together than either of them alone. Together, they offer a map for a full spectrum of healing and thriving from the darkest and most unconscious places within us.

THE POWER OF STORY

This book weaves research, theory, and lived experiences—my own and those of others I have counseled, taught, and corresponded with for more than two decades. When sharing stories from my own life, the details are true and accurate, except when I have altered the particulars in order to protect someone's identity. The stories involving clients and readers are also real but are often presented as composites to protect confidentiality. So if you identify with any particular story while you're reading this and suspect that I am referring to you, I assure you that I'm not. Our struggles, even when hidden, resound with others across the globe.

I hold the unbroken confidentiality of hundreds of people who struggle to reconcile and integrate their deep spiritual insights and aspirations with their traumas, shadowy aspects of their psyche, and gritty challenges of being human. When I published my fourth book, *Halfway Up the Mountain: The Error of Premature Claims to Enlightenment,* in 1999, I began to hear poignant stories of disillusionment and struggle that occur within various spiritual communities. I continued to hear these stories as I wrote two more books on spirituality and psychology: *Eyes Wide Open: Cultivating Discernment on the Spiritual Path* in 2009 and *The Guru Question: The Perils and Rewards of Choosing a Spiritual Teacher* in 2011. The subsequent outpouring of personal accounts of dignified struggles through trauma and scandal were heartbreaking. Although each version was unique, most of these stories included familiar themes, patterns, and repetitions. One of the most common refrains was some version of: *I realize now that I had unconsciously hoped that yoga (or my spiritual path) would take away my emotional and existential suffering, yet no matter how many years of yoga and meditation I do, my struggles and challenges haven't gone away.*

I share stories like this here so that you will remember that you are not alone. By recognizing our shared humanity, we can release the shame and secrecy we have been carrying throughout our lives, and we can even avoid falling into the profound suffering that others have experienced by learning from their accounts. We can also gain motivation and fortitude by drawing upon the tremendous successes and psychological transformations of others.

NOW WE BEGIN AGAIN

The first of Patanjali's Yoga Sutras says *Atha Yoga Anushasanam*—"Now we begin again." Whether we have been traveling the path of self-knowledge for decades or have just begun the conscious journey, we choose to begin again now and forever. Recognizing ourselves as fellow travelers on the journey, each gifted with irreplaceable gifts and highly personal labyrinths to traverse, we humbly avail ourselves of the extraordinary paths that have been laid before us, and we commit ourselves to becoming unique embodiments of these fields of knowledge and expression.

The rising wave of integration has increased in momentum and now wants to break free. It wants yoga to be "populated" with Western psychology and Western psychology to be infused with yoga and other somatic-oriented spiritual traditions. As we evolve in this direction together, we create a wellspring of information, wisdom, and practice that people from around the world can both contribute to and drink from. When we practice this integration in our own lives and share it with others, its positive effects ripple out into the larger world. I have trained people who bring this work to firefighters, law enforcement officials, prisons, hospitals, schools, trauma and treatment centers, and juvenile-detention facilities. As you read this book, I invite you to consider your own brand of offering the synthesis of yoga and psychology.

If possible, I invite you to intentionally engage with the practices offered herein for a minimum of two to three months. Try on what you are reading, dive into the practices you resonate with, and apply them to your personal practice and to those in your sphere of influence. Several of these practices are short and have relevance to almost any population. Once you've learned them, you can practice them throughout the day and on the fly. When we bring the brilliance of yoga and psychology together in a directly personal way, we immediately partake in their integrated abundance. And because the knowledge we awake arises within our own body, deep psyche, and spirit, there is no end to the possibilities for growth and deepening.

The cultivation of this field belongs to none of us, and it is available to us all. It beckons us into its open arms to collectively contribute to its evolution. With folded hands and flowers, I offer this book to you, my readers.

PART I

THE BIRTH
OF A FIELD

1

THE MARRIAGE OF
ANCIENT WISDOM AND
DEPTH PSYCHOLOGY

Out beyond ideas of wrongdoing and rightdoing, there is a field. I'll meet you there," wrote the thirteenth-century poet Rumi. This book is an invitation to create a new field in which we discover the endless mysteries of yoga and the deep psyche—a place to practice deeply with these exquisite, complementary inner traditions. Doing so as a globally linked community, we can collaborate, co-create, exchange knowledge and skills, and together become more than any of us can be alone.

Whether you are a yoga teacher or psychologist, a student of either practice, a health professional, or simply someone who wants to explore themselves and these subjects, you are entering a field in which anyone with sincerity and interest can find a place. You, the reader, are an essential voice in the birth of this field. Picking up this book indicates a curiosity—and most likely some experience or expertise—in one or both of these fields. Together we are engaging in a collective inquiry, investigation, dialogue, and exploration into this intersection of disciplines. By allowing psychology to impact yoga, and yoga to influence psychology, they each become more through the inclusion of the other—and we become more through the inclusion of each other's wisdom and alliance. Once you gain the foundation presented in this book,

I encourage you to engage in your own experiments, theories, research, and practices, and to contribute to this evolving field.

⚛

Psychology is a field in the making. Whereas the yoga tradition is estimated to be anywhere from 2,500 to 5,000 years old, Western psychology has been a recognizable field for only about 135 years.[1] Globalization, increased interest on the part of Westerners in Eastern spirituality, and significant developments in neuroscience, trauma research, and somatic psychology all have opened the doors for a truly new synthesis of Eastern and Western approaches to mental, physical, and spiritual health.

Sri Aurobindo (1872–1950)—an Indian nationalist, philosopher, and yoga master—taught that the desire for a transcendent, beyond-this-world enlightenment found in various spiritual traditions needed to be turned inward, or involuted, in order to transform our bodies at a cellular level and positively affect society on a grander level. I also believe this to be true and imperative at this time of environmental and political intensity. We who are interested in greater possibilities are not called to merely transcend the life we live and the earth we inhabit, but to transform them.

Part of this evolution includes transmuting the psychological aspect of our experience. We need to understand our own psychology in a deep way, penetrating our conditioning and understanding its multigenerational influence on us, and transforming unconscious limitations and conditioned ideas of who we are and how we are to live. Doing so, we become free to fully apply the great truths that yoga and other spiritual traditions have to offer. When that occurs, we increase our ability to penetrate our psychology more fully, which further opens spiritual awareness that again bears upon psychological deepening. In this way, we create a golden thread of infinity as to the possibilities of psychological and spiritual unfolding.

I envision a field of yoga in which more and more people of various backgrounds, cultures, ages, life stages, body types, and degrees

4

of health and illness engage with this extraordinary practice that has thrived for thousands of years. I also envision a quality of yoga practiced in the Western world that embraces the value that psychological insight has to offer teachers and practitioners. In this way, people can simultaneously heal physically and psychologically and, if they wish, explore the deeper spiritual insights of yoga, which become more accessible through the tools of psychology.

YOGA: THE ENDLESS EXPANSE

As I mentioned before, the precise origins of yoga are not known, and even renowned yoga scholars disagree on the historical dates of its inception. Writer and philosopher Mircea Eliade suggests that the first systematized form of yoga could have been written by Patanjali in his Yoga Sutras sometime between 300 BCE and 500 CE.[2] Georg Feuerstein proposes that less structured yogic ideas and practices can be found dating back to the time of the Rig Veda, a Hindu text and hymns composed before 1900 BCE.[3] India religion scholar Edwin Bryant, PhD, asserts there are images of figures in yogic postures dating as far back as 3000 BCE.[4]

Throughout the course of this book, when I refer to yoga, I'm not just talking about the physical postures that yoga is commonly associated with in the Western world. I'm referring to everything yoga entails—asana, meditation, breathwork, ethics, self-care, service to the world, concepts of consciousness, and views on personal development. Looking at yoga from this wider perspective, we discover many of the goals of modern psychology to be complementary with those of yoga. Yet what yoga distinctly offers are maps of consciousness that expand far beyond where most psychology ends. These maps can add enormous depth, richness, and valuable tools to Western psychological approaches. Additionally, they're more accessible than the interpretations of consciousness offered by other spiritual traditions. Unlike contemporary religions that offer a viewpoint that adherents are expected to believe and follow at face value, yoga offers practices that introduce direct, personal experience of what it teaches.

Even if you have decades of yogic practice, you will continue to encounter new subtleties, blind spots, pitfalls, challenges, and unforeseen possibilities along the path. Fortunately, the yogic masters have already mapped these out in incredible detail. If you soar into the domains of angels, yoga has already mapped out how to navigate that territory. If you fall from grace, yoga offers guidelines to pick yourself up again. No matter how deep you immerse yourself in yogic practice, no matter how far your consciousness expands, yoga will give you a map to guide the way. But yoga doesn't ask you to mistake the map for the journey itself. Yoga shows you the way and expects you to experiment and make your own discoveries. Yoga teaches us to experience spirituality for ourselves, as opposed to just taking someone else's word for it.

The physical practice of asana is so effective and timeless that it translates into every culture in which it is placed. We are living in a time in which yoga is literally taking root in new countries and populations with unprecedented frequency. A 2016 study conducted by *Yoga Journal* and Yoga Alliance reveals that there are nearly 37 million yoga practitioners in the United States (up from 20.4 million in 2012), and 34 percent of Americans say they are "somewhat or very likely" to practice yoga in the next year (the equivalent of more than 80 million Americans). The study also shows that 37 percent of practitioners have children younger than eighteen who also practice yoga.[5] These days, there seem to be few people who disagree with the value of yoga. It shows up in all types of places: organizations that serve veterans, the elderly, youth, and underprivileged populations of every kind; businesses; government; conventional and alternative medicine practices; insurance companies; the corporate world; centers for trauma and conflict resolution; and among the millions of people who find a spiritual or inner connection and increased physical and mental health through its practices.

There's a common fallacy that people need to be flexible, young, or physically fit to do yoga. The reality is that anyone can practice. In my teaching experience, even students who are highly compromised in terms of physical capacity still benefit from yoga. One student could not engage in physical movement without overheating, so I helped him follow the yoga instructions mentally, visualizing the practice and working with his breath. He gained immense physical and emotional benefits from the practice. Of the 196 *sutras*, or idioms, that comprise the Yoga Sutras, only three refer to the physical practice of asana. Although many people prefer to enter the yogic path through asana, yoga also offers doorways of breathing techniques, meditation, and internal practices available to people at every age and stage of development.

Yoga is a popular complement to the practices of other spiritual traditions, and you'll find yoga as a component of religious retreats around the world. People from all backgrounds enjoy yoga without feeling that doing so contradicts the teachings of their traditions. Buddhists have been incorporating yoga into their seated and walking meditation practices, and people from all backgrounds practice *kirtan* or attend concerts to hear the sacred chants. Once, in Barcelona, I sang *mantras* with hundreds of people at an outdoor gathering. In Israel, I was exposed to the Om Shalom movement, which integrates the physical practices of yoga with the prayers and philosophical teachings of Judaism.

Big business—particularly in the fields of fashion design, physical fitness, and nutrition—has taken note of yoga's popularity, often to the dismay of committed yogic practitioners. The 2016 study conducted by *Yoga Journal* and Yoga Alliance mentioned earlier states that the "annual practitioners' spending on yoga classes, clothing, equipment, and accessories rose to $16 billion, up from $10 billion over the past four years."[6] Yoga has also become popular among professional athletes and is marketed to fans of those sports, including professional football, surfing, and mixed martial arts, to name a few. Whereas many serious practitioners feel concerned that this "dumbing down" and commercialization of yoga confuses people about the real nature of yoga, others believe that entering the practice of yoga at any level still brings benefit and offers a doorway to discovering yoga's deeper dimensions.

PSYCHE: THE ENDLESS INTERIOR

Psyche refers to a concept of the intangible self. Although the self is invisible, it is felt palpably within all of us. Originating from Latin and Greek, the term refers to "the soul, mind, spirit; breath; life, one's life, the invisible animating principle or entity which occupies and directs the physical body; understanding."[7] I choose to use the term *psyche* because it intimates centuries of thought regarding the self and soul prior to the somewhat recent construction of the field of psychology. Specifically, *psyche* points to an aspect of the human being that is individual, unique, more unconscious than conscious, and conditioned through time, yet capable of transformation.

In contrast to the infinite expanse of yoga, Western psychology—in particular somatic psychology, trauma research, and neuroscience—has discovered methods to unravel and heal the ailments that afflict the Western psyche while valuing the individual's unique personal story and history. I choose to address the Western psyche in this book rather than the global psyche because individual cultures impact the structure and formation of the human psyche. As a Western psychologist, I have worked successfully with people from different cultures throughout the world, and it is my hope that the proposed integration of yoga and psychology will be relevant to people of other cultures. However, I also want to be clear about the limits of my knowledge of the formation of the psyche in cultures far different from my own.

Carl Jung (1875–1961) was one of the first Western psychologists to make the connection between psyche and yoga, and he articulated some of the most eloquent thoughts on the psyche itself. Although not always known as such, Jung was a modern mystic who explored the esoteric domains of consciousness, including the vast territory of the unconscious, in a way similar to that of the yogis. However, Jung valued and embraced the personal and archetypal dimensions of the human being that yogis have often ignored or prematurely transcended. He spent much of his life exploring the experiences, images, desires, and longings of humans everywhere. In his *Psychology and Religion: East and West*, Jung writes, "I would not advise anyone to touch yoga without careful analysis of his unconscious reaction."[8] Although we as a culture have come a long way from this perspective, this statement points to Jung's respect for the power of the deeper dimensions of yoga.

In *Civilization in Transition*, Jung asserts, "Even if the whole world were to fall to pieces, the unity of the psyche would never be shattered. And the wider and more numerous the fissures on the surface, the more the unity is strengthened in the depths."[9] Some Eastern traditions regard the psyche and psychology from an impersonal perspective, suggesting that "life is but a dream," and they view the psyche as something unreal and impenetrable, and something to be transcended. Jung and his contemporaries, however, offered a doorway to the nascent field of spiritualized psychology. Unlike others, they held a deep respect for the psyche and recognized the value of exploring it, relating to it, and discovering an inherently spiritual process of unfolding by doing so.

In my own explorations, I have found the psyche to have an invisible but palpable "shape" that can almost be seen. It can be molded, worked with, and moved into healthier, deeper, and more integrated shapes, bringing people more happiness. As a young psychologist, and particularly during my early forays into spirituality as a late teen, the psyche seemed like an impossible labyrinth to engage with, much less unwind. Yet over the years I have found I can engage with it and help it transform into its full potential, and this particularly happens when combining Western psychology with yogic practices. With dedication, time, and skillful guidance, even a tangled psychological makeup can be unwoven and transformed.

Western psychology also offers interest in—and inclusion of—the shadow elements we all have within us. These are aspects of ourselves that we repress from awareness but that often cause pain or even harm to ourselves and those around us. The shadow is somewhat accounted for in yogic teachings as an aspect of the unconscious mind that one aims to transcend, or it is worked with meditatively through yogic deities. However, in Western psychology, the shadow is the gateway to integrating aspects of the unconscious in order to become a more unified and individuated human being. In *Modern Man in Search of a Soul*, Jung writes:

In contrast to the meditation found in yoga practice, the psychoanalytic aim is to observe the shadowy presentation—whether in the form of images or of feelings—that are spontaneously evolved in the unconscious psyche and appear without his bidding to the [person] who looks within. In this way we find once more things that we have repressed or forgotten. Painful though it may be, this is in itself a gain—for what is inferior or even worthless belongs to me as my Shadow and gives me substance and mass. How can I be substantial if I fail to cast a Shadow? I must have a dark side also if I am to be whole; and inasmuch as I become conscious of my Shadow, I also remember that I am a human being like any other.[10]

YOGA AND PSYCHOLOGY RESEARCH

Science matters. And it is particularly valuable when examining the integration of yoga and Western psychology because research can promote the acceptance of yoga and its practice in tandem with psychology into mainstream policy, thus linking contemporary science with sincere spiritual practice. Fortunately, yoga has recently been widely studied through the lens of scientific research, and thus the intuition of the yogic mystics is now supported through science in a way that is beginning to bring it into mainstream acceptance and helping it garner public funding.

My research for this book is an overview of the popular literature related to this subject, as well as an outline of the academic research done to date on the integration of yoga with psychology and its related fields. A team of five talented graduate-school interns and I included studies on yoga's impact on stress, as well as the use of yoga in treating clinical diagnoses and promoting well-being. We also researched yoga and neuroscience literature, studies regarding the usage of yoga to treat trauma, and investigations into the integration of yoga and somatic psychology. From approximately two hundred studies, we developed the following propositions:

1. The Western psychologist can benefit from insights, practices, and research on yoga.

2. The Western practitioner of yoga can benefit by integrating the larger yogic perspective of breathwork and meditation, as well as somatic psychology, neuroscience, trauma research, mindfulness, and other developments in Western psychology.

3. The long-term integration of these two fields offers the practitioner the possibility of becoming fully embodied— for the consciousness and intelligence that are ordinarily associated with the mind to become awakened throughout the whole body.

4. There is a new field emerging in which a variety of methods that integrate yoga and psychology can be created, researched, and implemented.

There is ample evidence to show that yoga has a positive effect on post-traumatic stress disorder (PTSD), depression, anxiety, immunity issues, eating disorders, attention deficit hyperactivity disorder (ADHD), schizophrenia, well-being, and mood. More than 150 detailed references for the studies cited below are available online in an article published in the *Journal of Transpersonal Psychology* entitled "Yoga Psychotherapy: The Integration of Western Psychological Theory and Ancient Yogic Wisdom."[11] Here are some highlights:

Yoga Reduces Stress

"Yoga for Anxiety and Depression," an article in the *Harvard Mental Health Letter*, addresses the significance of yoga on stress management. It asserts that by "reducing perceived stress and anxiety, yoga appears to modulate stress response systems. This, in turn, decreases physiological arousal—for example, reducing the heart rate, lowering blood pressure, and easing respiration. There is also evidence that yoga practices help increase heart-rate variability, an indicator of the body's ability to respond to stress with more flexibility."[12] Additional studies have found the following:

- A relationship exists between yoga and decreased stress in young adults, older adults, businesswomen and men, and patients suffering from chronic illness.

- Yoga has the ability to train the body to relax on a muscular level, helping practitioners to more easily manage their stress response.

- Compared to beginners, advanced practitioners of physical yoga displayed lower levels of stress and increased awareness of being present in the moment.

- Yoga helps adults and traumatized youth regulate their emotions and practice self-soothing techniques.

- Yoga's meditative practices and breathwork (pranayama) have been shown to promote emotional regulation.

Yoga Can Assist in Treating Clinical Diagnoses

Yoga has been shown to assist children with a diagnosis of attention deficit hyperactivity disorder (ADHD). Specifically, yoga practice has been used to help them stabilize their emotions, reduce hyper-activity and impulsivity, increase attention span, provide feelings of calmness and confidence, and improve social skills. Yoga also has been shown to improve sleep patterns, parent-child relationships, and the child's approach to school.[13]

People who suffer from eating disorders and also practice yoga have experienced improved mood, increased physical and emotional awareness, and decreased symptoms of their disorders. Overeating and "emotional eating" were also reduced. One study reported that through yoga "women's intense fear of gaining weight, preoccupation with weight, body dissatisfaction, extreme desire to be thinner, and desire to think about and engage in bouts of binge eating was reduced."[14] Again, when yoga is practiced in conjunction with effective psychotherapy, a far more holistic approach to treatment becomes available.

Yoga has also been shown to benefit those who suffer from schizophrenia by reducing symptoms of psychopathology when paired with standard psychiatric treatment. Studies have also found yoga to reduce psychotic symptoms and depression, improve cognition, enhance social and occupational functioning, and increase quality of life.[15]

There is a large body of scientific data that demonstrates yoga's capacity to decrease depression and anxiety, which are often associated with each other. One study asserted that women diagnosed with major depressive disorder who were assigned to a yoga intervention group showed a decrease in depression and experienced less rumination, increased feelings of connectedness, and the added benefit of a new coping method.[16] Another study concluded that yoga's ability to calm the nervous system, foster an awareness of the present moment, and release energy trapped in the body aided in the reduction of symptoms associated with affective disorders.[17]

In addition, studies show that the practice of following the breath, found in both yoga and in Buddhist mindfulness practices, is a valuable support in the treatment of depression and anxiety. One study found that diaphragmatic yogic breathing increases ego strength, emotional stability, confidence, alertness, and perceived control over one's environment, and reduces anxiety, depression, phobic behavior, and psychosomatic problems.[18] Another group researched how the suppression of inner experiences, possibly triggered by traumatic events, may be linked to inhibited breathing, which in turn may worsen states of depression and anxiety.[19]

Amy Weintraub, a yoga teacher with a wide background in psychology, has written extensively on how yoga practices can be used to treat depression and anxiety, specifically in her books *Yoga Skills for Therapists* and *Yoga for Depression*. Weintraub instructs therapists to learn and teach a variety of yogic techniques—including those focused on breath, sound, *mudras* (hand positions), imagery, and self-inquiry—to increase the effectiveness of psychotherapy.

Yoga Promotes Well-Being

Even those who do not suffer from diagnosable psychological disorders can experience boosts in general well-being through yoga. In one study, healthy participants recorded the fluctuations of their mood and emotional states before and after yoga classes. The results showed that positive moods increased and negative moods decreased following their practice.[20] Other research compared the benefits of walking to yoga practice and found that those who were assigned to the yoga group reported greater improvements in both mood and anxiety than those in the walking group.[21] Yoga practice additionally promotes greater well-being by increasing body awareness, positive affect (mood), and life satisfaction for both men and women, while simultaneously decreasing objectification of their bodies.[22]

Yoga can also provide a space for connection and relationship building. Partner-oriented yoga can foster emotional connection, healthy boundaries, trust, and a strong sense of self while simultaneously being in relationship, according to recent research.[23] Various forms of doing yoga with other people include AcroYoga, which combines partner yoga, acrobatics, community building, and play, offering participants a joyful and therapeutic form of engagement; and Laughter Yoga, which is designed to promote joy through a communal experience of shared laughter.

The ability to be present increases with the practice of yoga, and an emerging field of research has shown that mindfulness practices help people increase attention and focus.[24] Another study found that just eight weeks of yoga practice significantly increased mindfulness, insightful understanding, and an open attitude.[25] Psychiatrist Mark Epstein, MD, has published a number of articles detailing how meditation is useful in exploring issues of personality and maturity among relatively healthy individuals.[26] Findings such as these are important to consider when thinking about preventive mental health, protecting against anxiety and depression, and strengthening the existing resources that each individual possesses.

Furthermore, advances in neuroscience validate and offer new data to support the value of yoga's contribution to psychological well-being. For example, research shows that practicing mindfulness meditation increases positive affect and enhances self-regulation.[27] Certain areas of the brain associated with attention, introspection, and sensory processing are more prominent in participants with extensive meditation experience compared to those with little to no experience.

THE MIGRATION OF YOGA FROM EAST TO WEST

As an aspect of Hinduism, yoga represents one of the most effective importations and migrations of a contemporary world religion that has occurred in recent history. Yoga has moved seamlessly wherever it is imported, not only from East to West, but also throughout Central and South America, Asia, Africa, the Middle East, and virtually everywhere else around the world.[28]

Swami Vivekananda, a renowned teacher from India, spoke at the 1893 Parliament of World Religions in Chicago. He proposed greater exchange between Eastern and Western spiritual traditions and began his speech with the salutation, "Sisters and brothers of America," and was immediately met with a standing ovation. In 1951, Bengali philosopher Haridas Chaudhuri received the blessing of his guru, the Indian revolutionary Sri Aurobindo, to come to San Francisco, where he planted the seeds for what became the California Institute of Integral Studies, the first East-West accredited graduate school (where I studied and taught for years). In 1962, Esalen Institute was founded by Michael Murphy and Richard Price as a laboratory to bring together cutting-edge developments in the human-potential field by both Eastern and Western traditions. In 1966, Yogi Amrit Desai created the Kripalu Center for Yoga and Health, the largest yoga center in the United States, which to this day continues offering innovative programs in yoga and psychology. These are but a few of the key figures and organizations who formed the foundation for this historically unprecedented migration of yoga from East to West, presenting new possibilities for a global interchange of knowledge and traditions.

As I noted before, most of the Western world's interest in yoga is limited to physical postures. I believe this comes from the accessibility and effectiveness of posture practice, but also because a lot of yoga's philosophical origins have been lost in importation. Even so, more people are becoming interested in the other aspects of yoga, specifically meditation, and those who enter through the door of physical yoga practice often find themselves immersed in a deeper yogic journey than they originally thought possible.

I received a Facebook "friend" request from a young man doing Tree Pose on a wooden dugout canoe in Sierra Leone, West Africa. I asked him where he learned yoga, and he told me that one of my good friends, Veronica Geretz, had brought yoga to Sierra Leone while completing her graduate-school internship in peace studies. Today, people gather there in a small studio to practice. This story struck a chord in me, as I palpably felt the spread of yoga throughout the world through individuals who love and resonate with the practice.

Jung coined the term *gnostic intermediary* to describe someone who can "personally incorporate the wisdom of a tradition and can then speak directly from their own experience and translate this experience and understanding into the language and concepts of the culture to which they wish to communicate."[29] Because yoga integrates easily with other traditions, ordinary practitioners become gnostic intermediaries as they translate yoga into their lives, regardless of the contexts of era, religion, and culture. The successful importation of yoga into Western and worldwide culture, and its effective integration with psychology, will come from people who practice in their own lives while simultaneously "holding hands" at a fundamental level and practicing together.

Years ago, I attended an event where my Sufi mentor and friend, Llewellyn Vaughan-Lee, was teaching with a well-known shaman to explore the relationship between Sufism and shamanism. A sincere young practitioner in the back raised his hand and said, "All of this awareness and depth of connection is accessible when I meditate here, but when I am practicing alone in my house . . ." At that point, Llewellyn interrupted him and lovingly but firmly asserted, "You are *never* meditating alone. You are always meditating with these people and many more all over the world." I never forgot that. Llewellyn insisted that we consider that we actually live on a *planet*, not just in a particular country, and that we remember we are intertwined with the natural world and each other. Even when we feel alone, we are truly interconnected.

As yoga continues to grow in the West, I also want to explore what the West can contribute to the evolution of yoga. What can happen when yoga integrates the best of Western psychology, specifically that pertaining to somatic treatments, trauma recovery, and neuroscience? This unfolding inquiry is alive throughout this book. Stephen Cope, a psychologist and yoga teacher, wrote in *Yoga and the Quest for the True Self*:

> The point of intersection that I describe is fascinating not only because of the capacity the ancient science of yoga has to change our lives, but also because of the capacity we have to change yoga. Through its intersection with the West, yoga is undergoing a time of enormous evolution. It is being feminized, democratized, and brought into relationship with contemporary medicine, Western psychology, and with Buddhism, Judaism, and Christianity.[30]

It's amazing to consider the vast cultural exchange occurring today, its future implications, and our unique role in the process. I believe we do have a responsibility, depending upon how widely we represent the yogic teachings, to make sure that essential aspects of yoga do not get "lost in translation." This is why the best yoga teachers develop their knowledge of yoga throughout their lives. Doing so enables us to remain close to yoga's philosophical and mystical origins as we move forward and integrate it with contemporary psychology and science. And, as

I've asserted before, I believe that Western psychology is the key to help us unlock the multiple doors of yoga's depths, clearing psychological blocks to our permeability to its ancient teachings—including its focus on breath, meditation, visualization, and other esoteric practices.

Yoga and psychology are like perfect lovers. Each is distinct and uniquely valuable, but when they join they create endless possibilities for transformation that are far greater than what is available when either is practiced alone. When we unite the brilliance of these two streams, the potential is truly endless, particularly when the integrated wisdom arises in one's body, psyche, and spirit. Yoga and psychology together form a seamless weave of knowledge and practices applicable in whatever moment we find ourselves—whether in the yoga studio, in the therapist's office, or in any of the activities that life may bring.

2

WHY YOGA NEEDS
PSYCHOLOGY

There was a flood tide of nearly incomprehensible
Hindu metaphysics, filled with high-flown descriptions
of ecstatic states . . . But where were the descriptions of
neurotic Western seekers like myself? Where was my story?
STEPHEN COPE, *Yoga and the Quest for the True Self*[1]

It's *not* all good!" shouted my Ashtanga teacher Bhavani Maki. She was addressing a collection of local surfers, hippy travelers, famous locals, affluent vacationers, and serious yoga students in attendance at her morning class in Kaua'i, Hawai'i. "In fact, some of it just plain sucks! No matter how much yoga you do"—her voice softened—"or how many times you hear the locals say, 'It's all good,' and how many times you tell yourself that, it just isn't. Shit happens."

Everyone in the room knew she was right. Deep down inside, nobody really believes "It's all good" all of the time. Difficult emotions, human interactions, and experiences arise for each of us on a daily basis. We may tell ourselves or want to believe that yoga or meditation will eventually remove our suffering and perhaps even bring us to enlightenment, but it just doesn't happen that way for most people. Sustained yoga practice can provide enormous benefit some of the time, but the rest of the time we are simply human, and there is no escape from that no matter who we are, novice or master. All lives include joy and suffering, sickness and health, grief and renewal, tragedy and ecstasy.

THE WOUNDS OF THE WESTERN PSYCHE

Even though yoga is now practiced widely in the Western world, it was created in an Eastern culture with psyches quite different from our own. There is a tendency in both Eastern and Western teachers of yoga to claim that its philosophies and practices provide everything we need to transform our lives as Western practitioners. This might prove true for some people, but the vast majority of practitioners and teachers will never have the time, guidance, or support it takes to integrate and translate the esoteric practices of yoga into their Western psychological makeup. Furthermore, I believe it is not optimal to do so. A friend of mine once asked the Dalai Lama if she could become a Buddhist nun and put on the robes of a renunciant in order to immerse herself in practice. "You can," he told her, "but in twenty years you will probably take them off." He then explained that she would need to integrate the Buddhist teachings into her own cultural context at some point.

To understand why Western psychology has so much to contribute to yoga, it is important to realize that yoga was created in a highly specific cultural context with particular variables. To begin with, the physical postures that the Western world largely identifies as "yoga" were brought to popularity in India by men: B. K. S. Iyengar, K. Pattabhi Jois, and T. K. V. Desikachar, among others. Although the vast majority of yoga practitioners are women, the earlier importations of yoga into the Western world were taught in a masculine form suited to masculine bodies, with a focus on rigor, power, and stamina. This style of yoga did not take into account women's bodies and the specific ways that women (and the feminine aspects of all of us) are best attended to and transformed.

Second, yoga alone rarely addresses common afflictions in Western culture: trauma, anxiety, depression, loneliness, self-esteem and self-worth issues, grief, difficult relationships and longing for relationships, parenting problems, wounding and/or isolation from our biological family of origin, addiction, codependence, and other challenges that Westerners struggle with at some point in their lives. Whereas yoga does provide tools to address suffering in a global way, it does not provide the detail and precision that Western psychology offers.

PSYCHOLOGY AND CONSCIOUSNESS

Psychology is all in the details. It addresses the *contents* of consciousness, whereas yoga focuses on the *context* of consciousness. Yoga addresses our unity as human beings and the structures of consciousness and workings of ego that transcend cultural and individual distinctions, but psychology takes into account our differences and diversity. In psychology, the story we have about our lives matters, including our unique gifts and inevitable human sufferings. Our individuality and the unconscious patterns that run large aspects of our lives are not prematurely transcended, but embraced and illuminated. As Carl Jung wrote, "One does not become enlightened by imagining figures of light, but by making the darkness conscious. The latter process is disagreeable and therefore not popular."[2]

Some schools of yoga suggest that psychology is useless, unspiritual, a waste of time, and even a narcissistic indulgence of the illusory ego. Teachers who think this way discourage their students from psychological exploration, suggesting it is an endless labyrinth that goes nowhere and simply reinforces the nature of the false self. They describe the world of the psyche as *maya*, which is loosely (and, in my opinion, ineffectively) translated as "illusion."

"Life is but a dream," these yoga teachers assert. Or they quickly remind us that our goal is to get off the "wheel of karma." I was given this message directly when I lived in an ashram during my twenties. My friend Laura and I often hid in the woods and shared our confusion about such teachings. "I don't want to get off the wheel," she would say. "Yeah, I like being alive and want to come back," I'd respond.

Over time, I have come to a more nuanced understanding of these principles, largely informed by the tantric teachings from both Hindu and Buddhist traditions. It was the late yogic scholar Georg Feuerstein who suggested to me that maya didn't mean that life was an illusion but rather that it referred to our "illusory relationship to life." Therefore the practices of yoga and psychology are about clarifying our confused relationship to ourselves and all of life rather than trying to transcend it. Deep psychology endeavors to make the unconscious conscious by "enlightening" the dark or unconscious forces within us.

Teachers of yoga and other Eastern traditions who espouse the above view do not typically possess experience or training in psychology. Psychology is relatively new, and some of its most notable advances (neuroscience, trauma research, and somatics, specifically) are only decades old. Additionally, when it comes to depth practices like yoga and psychology, there is no substitute for doing introspective work. I have often heard teachers of yoga say things like, "I haven't actually been to therapy but I talk with wise friends," or, "Many of my friends are therapists so talking to them is like going to therapy." On the contrary, there is no replacement for actually working on the contents of one's psyche under the guidance of a skillful psychotherapist. Some people imagine that if they open the door to their interior that they will be overwhelmed with what they discover and perhaps have no way to cope with it. Indeed, without skillful help this can happen. Some people consciously and unconsciously choose to keep the door to their deep psyche closed and their awareness limited and superficial, while others try to transcend their inner psychological experience through yoga and other spiritual practices. I'll talk about this more in the next section. However, psychology gives a language for the unconscious and teaches people to communicate about it effectively.

For those who are deeply committed to the psychological path, it is a monumental discovery to experience the psyche as workable. It is malleable and penetrable, and we can learn to work with it, rather than allowing it to control us. I have come to understand this with total conviction after more than twenty years of experience in the field. The degree to which we gain understanding and fluency with our own psyche depends largely upon the extent to which we engage with our investigation and on the quality of teachings, mentors, and tools we're exposed to.

For some, access to psychological tools to alleviate shame, to increase self-esteem, and to address anxiety, depression, addiction, and relationship issues can be sufficiently life changing. Yet for others (as we'll see in chapter 4), inquiry into the psyche becomes a profound path of self-discovery that is limitless in the best sense of the word. Often compared to an ocean that may appear calm or wavy on the surface, the psyche illuminates greater subtlety and unfolds endless inner depths the further we dive into it.

SPIRITUAL BYPASSING

I once visited an old friend in France who had run a yoga studio for years and had an advanced practice of Ashtanga Yoga—a rigorous and powerful form of physical posture practice. She told me that she had realized that although she had done a highly advanced and physically demanding practice of yoga almost every single day for years, she discovered that she had not really *been* there. She was engaging her physical body, yet at the same time was completely spaced out and not connected with her embodied, emotional, and psychological experience. She realized that decades of yoga had not brought her any closer to her emotions. Upon that recognition, she began psychotherapy and was processing old issues surrounding her feelings of abandonment and rejection as a result of being adopted. She had also begun an intimate, positive, and happy romantic relationship for the first time in years. She shifted her approach to yoga practice to something softer, slower, and more connected to the emotional aspects of her embodied experience.

Spiritual bypassing, a term coined by the American Buddhist psychologist John Welwood, refers to the ways that people use spiritual ideas and practices to avoid or prematurely transcend psychological wounds, weak ego structures, and low self-esteem in order to diminish personal needs, feelings, and developmental tasks in the name of spirituality or enlightenment. Spiritual bypassing is the process by which the egoic mechanism uses yoga and other practices to unconsciously circumvent—rather than work through—wounded, confused, and damaged aspects of our psyche. Spiritual bypassing

operates at all levels of spiritual development, from beginning practitioners to advanced yogis and spiritual masters. Access to spiritual
knowledge, when not integrated, can result in us fooling ourselves
that we are more evolved than we are. Although it is important that
we feel empowered by the hard-earned knowledge we have gained,
any notion of having "arrived" can impede further spiritual growth.
If we are in a position of spiritual authority or a transmitter of the
yoga tradition—which all yoga teachers are, whether they perceive
themselves to be or not—our unexamined spiritual bypassing is
likely to carry over into our yoga room.

I have encountered spiritual bypassing frequently in Western yoga.
People get drawn to yoga as a path that promises a foretold "enlightenment" as an escape from their suffering. It teaches a "big picture"
philosophy that gives people access to perspectives and practices that
temporarily alleviate their suffering—at least while in the yoga room.
Asana and breath practice offer a quick and organic high, and the
more we do of them, the higher we get. Again, there is nothing wrong
with this in and of itself, but the question is what do we do when we
come down from the high? I cannot underscore the hundreds of times
I have heard stories of frustrated yogis who access states of wellness,
peace, and equanimity during yoga but who lose it all within minutes
of leaving class.

Esoteric practices of yoga can elevate the diehard practitioner into
heightened states of consciousness for months or even years at a time,
becoming an addiction that is certainly healthier than drugs or alcohol,
but nonetheless is still a buffer to deeper emotional states. Although
yogic highs might be organic, the way we relate to them will dictate
when we are utilizing yoga to its fullest potential and when we are
employing yoga as a crutch or even an impediment to our development. If we are lucky, a good teacher, honest friend or colleague, or
romantic partner (if we can listen to their feedback) will let us know
that we are misusing our practice in this way. But when we use the
language of yogic dharma to buffer ourselves—as is so common in
spiritual bypassing—it takes an incredible amount of honesty and vulnerability to see through our own spiritualized defenses.

Some teachers and practitioners of yoga believe that if they truly throw themselves into spiritual practice that somehow their psychological challenges will dissipate in the light of awareness. There will always be someone promoting the idea that if we just follow our bliss and passion, our finances and practical circumstances will come together. Some people devote decades of their lives to spiritual practice yet remain emotionally underdeveloped. Well-known and respected teachers of yoga continue to privately wrestle with the reality that the awakening they experience—and perhaps even transmit to others—does not necessarily translate into more intimacy and happiness in their own lives, transform the difficult moments in their own relationships, make visible to themselves their blind spots, or keep anxiety and depression at bay. Most of these challenges belong to the domain of the psyche. Accordingly, they are most effectively worked with utilizing the tools of psychology and its developments.

Anything can be misused, including yoga. Some of my work as a psychotherapist involves a careful assessment of how the spiritual practices of my clients are serving their overall growth, as well as the ways they might be impeding or buffering them. In some cases, it is a matter of quantity; more is not always better. Sometimes people have to ease off on certain spiritual practices and attend more to psychological issues for a time in order to discover aspects of themselves that are unconscious or not addressed by the yogic practices they do. Excessively intense asana, mantra, and meditative practices that aim to transcend the body are examples of yogic practices that are frequently misused in the name of spiritual growth. Other times, we may have overemphasized certain aspects of our development and underemphasized others, and it is a question of rebalancing our efforts.

Given that spiritual bypassing is so common, how do we recognize it and work with it most effectively? Here is where psychological inquiry comes into play. After having humbly recognized the inevitability of spiritual bypassing and the reality that there is nothing wrong with it, we begin to understand the need to examine the psychological forces that run our lives far more than most of us would dare to imagine. Most of the psychologists and mystics I have interviewed assert that we are about 10 percent conscious and 90 percent unconscious. In other words, there is far more that we don't know about ourselves than we do.

Every human being has blind spots. When people say, "I know what my blind spots are," it always gives my head a little spin. By their very definition, they are blind—just like the blind spot we encounter on the road while driving. We may know those spots are there, but if we could see them while they were occurring they would not actually be obscured from our awareness. It is often in the context of relationship—ideally in a compassionate, supportive environment—that our blind spots can be most effectively seen and healed.

THE WOUNDS OF RELATIONSHIP REQUIRE RELATIONAL HEALING

Human beings are relational at their core. John Welwood suggests that "relational wounds" (the wounds that occur within human relationships) are most effectively healed in relationship with others.[3] People often assume that their core sufferings and traumas—many of which occurred in childhood and in various relational contexts throughout our lives—should be healed in the solitude of our own hearts and minds. Teachings of self-sufficiency and the dictate to meet one's own needs are often celebrated on the yogic path. I believe this is another way in which we use our spiritual ideas and practices to avoid the vulnerability of our humanity and our need for others to help us see ourselves, heal, and fulfill our needs for intimacy and community. Solo meditation practice and inner work are not often the most effective remedies to relational wounding. Therapeutic relationships, intimate relationships, close friendships, and spiritual mentorships can provide a context for healing that solo yogic and meditative practice cannot address in the same way.

Suzanne was a client of mine who experienced profound alienation and loneliness as a child. Her sincerity and concern about the environment, her preoccupation with death and other existential issues, and a desire to be of service at a young age were not understood or appreciated. She was repeatedly told that she thought too much. At a key moment in our therapy, after developing enough trust in our relationship, I was able to reflect to her the profound sincerity I saw in her and that I understood that as a child she was quite conscious and aware of the world around her and wanted to help. As she gently allowed my heartfelt reflection into her body, she shed tears of relief at having finally being seen and for the pain of having been missed by those around her as a child. In this recognition, Suzanne experienced a profound expansion of self-compassion that continued to grow throughout the months of our work. Suzanne had done spiritual practice for more than thirty years, yet it was only in relationship that this wound, which stemmed from a lack of psychological mirroring, could be touched and that specific aspects of healing could be accessed.

One of the benefits and motivating factors of the contemporary yoga class is that we practice within a group. People often express a wish to have more connection with those around them. One of the ways I address this desire is to have people introduce themselves to their neighbors in class or to include playful group poses. When I teach yoga intensives, I have people work together in dyads or small groups so they have an opportunity to share their personal experience. At lunch breaks during trainings, I try to create a context in which those who would like companionship can connect with others. All of us are vulnerable and everybody needs relationship, yet some people are more shy, introverted, or insecure. When the yoga teacher intentionally supports the need for relationship within the context of yoga, participants link yogic and psychological healing.

THE NEED TO ARTICULATE ONE'S INTENSITY

Arnaud Desjardins, the late French Advaita Vedanta master and documentary filmmaker, taught that every human being has a need to "articulate their intensity." He repeated this teaching during the years that I visited him, and it always struck a chord within me. When I lived in an ashram and was encouraged to transcend my personal story, something within me rebelled. Arnaud and his teacher, Swami

Prajnanpad of Northern India, were both adept with psychological knowledge. They taught that we must cross through the ocean of life in our pursuit toward spiritual heights and depths and learn to become one with all that arises, including all aspects of our experience.

Each human being, no matter who they are, has an intensity within them. Simply being alive, no matter our circumstance, brings with it a mental, emotional, physical, and often an existential intensity. The pervading truth of what the Buddhists call *impermanence*—the inevitable passing of everything that arises, particularly the inevitability of death—brings with it a certain intensity and profound vulnerability to every human experience. According to yogic philosophy, *prana*, or life force, animates each human body for the duration of their life and leaves at death. To be alive is to experience prana as it runs with intensity, vulnerability, and possibility through us.

Trauma, even in its everyday manifestations, can produce a lack of self-worth and self-esteem, as well as emptiness, sometimes repressing or numbing our inner intensity. Many people use vices like alcohol, drugs, excessive media, busyness, yoga, and other spiritual practice as buffers to our vulnerability. The human tendency to compare one's life to that of others can leave people believing that they lack importance or value, devaluing their own uniqueness, importance, and personal intensity. This is where psychology, with its recognition and appreciation for the importance of our personal narrative, becomes so relevant. We are not encouraged to transcend our experience, but to embody it.

The foundation of a rich therapeutic relationship is the capacity of the therapist to listen, empathize, and bring presence and unconditional acceptance to the client. Although this is but one aspect of psychotherapy, I am repeatedly amazed at the transformational power of listening and valuing another person. Sometimes those who are particularly shy or introverted need extra encouragement to recognize and give importance to their own inner intensity. It is as though through the therapist mirroring the client, he or she is able to recognize and value their intensity, uniqueness, and importance for the first time.

Once we recognize our own intensity, we come to understand and appreciate that everyone has it, no matter what their circumstances.

To express and receive our own and another's intensity is, as I noted in the previous section, a relational process and is not limited to the therapeutic relationship. It is something we can provide to each other. It requires us to recognize our own vulnerability and to allow it to be expressed in relationship to others.

WHY YOGA TEACHERS NEED PSYCHOLOGY AND PSYCHOTHERAPY

I have met numerous yoga teachers and dedicated practitioners who have a passionate interest in psychology but who do not want to undertake long-term studies in the subject. Some of them wish to bring a more nuanced psychological understanding into their own practice and teaching. Others are aware of the unexamined psychological content that may arise in the yoga room and don't know how to address and guide students through these processes.

Although yoga teachers are not licensed health-care professionals, issues of mental and physical health often emerge in the context of teaching yoga. The term *scope of practice* refers to the procedures, actions, and processes that a health-care practitioner is permitted to undertake in keeping with the terms of their professional license. The postures and breathing practices taught in yoga classes are powerful and often bring up strong emotional material, and it is not within the scope of practice of most yoga teachers to address these wounds. They are more effectively addressed in therapy and therapeutic groups led by professionals, or through pursuing more in-depth psychological and somatic training or the many new approaches to trauma-sensitive yoga.

Those who teach yoga as a profession inevitably come across students who are profoundly wounded and who want attention beyond the scope of the teacher's practice. This most often occurs when teachers offer intensives, teacher trainings, esoteric practices, or set themselves up (or are projected by their students to be) in a position of spiritual authority, but it can happen at any time. Accordingly, it is of utmost importance that yoga teachers understand the limits of their psychological capacity and have a list of resources that they can refer students to.

Furthermore, yoga teachers should understand the distinction between *neurosis* and *psychosis*—terms that are often used interchangeably without understanding the key distinction between them. Neurosis and psychosis exist on a spectrum in which the degree, duration, and resulting debilitation of symptoms distinguish the two. Neurosis refers to any mental or emotional imbalance that causes distress. We are all a little bit neurotic and experience imbalance at various times throughout our lives. The invisible line that occurs when our neurosis begins to impair our occupational, academic, or interpersonal functioning, either experienced by our own subjective experience or by those around us, is how *psychosis* or *psychopathology*—terms that can be used interchangeably—is determined.

The key manual that describes psychopathology in the disciplines of psychology and psychiatry is the *Diagnostic and Statistical Manual of Mental Disorders* (DSM-V), a thick volume that fortunately has a more accessible, condensed, desktop version, *Desk Reference to the Diagnostic Criteria from DSM-5*. The DSM is updated every several years to reflect developments in the field. When I teach courses in Yoga & Psyche, I recommend that students familiarize themselves with this resource—not so that they can diagnose people or become amateur psychologists, but so they have an understanding of some of the major forms of psychological challenges that are likely to arise in the yoga studio. Among the most common are anxiety and depressive disorders, a spectrum of eating disorders (many people with eating disorders are drawn to yoga), and mood disorders.

When I was in graduate school, we were required to take a class on psychopathology in order to understand the distinctions between the various types of psychosis and mental disorders that can occur. In retrospect, I remember fondly—at the time it was dead serious!—how each week one of us would come to class convinced that he or she had a severe form of psychopathology. The teacher would empathically help us to understand that in the process of self-discovery and psychological inquiry, we might discover aspects of these conditions in ourselves, but that psychosis was determined by the severity and duration of symptoms, which were often far more severe than most of us experienced.

Another important reason for teachers to engage in psychotherapy or psychological inquiry is to prevent spiritual scandals. Almost all such scandals happen due to the psychological blind spots in spiritual teachers *and* their students. It is not that the spiritual practices that they teach and practice are flawed, but that an equal depth of psychological self-awareness does not accompany them.

The challenges all people face—particularly those of us born into a world where trauma is not something that affects just a few individuals (as we will see in chapter 7)—are simply not going to be addressed by yoga alone. Again, the yoga of the East was not designed to address the psychological traumas of the West. When there is a crisis or scandal, no matter how many times we chant *Om*, or how many yogic practices we engage in, it is not going to heal our psychological and relational wounds. People need to heal, feel, talk, and work things through. They need to understand how they contributed to the dynamic, what they have learned, how to forgive themselves and others, and how to transform their pain. This is a place where psychology is so brilliant and irreplaceable in its capacity.

In my experience as a psychotherapist and researcher, I have arrived at the conclusion that about 80 to 90 percent of male spiritual teachers—and a strikingly smaller percentage of female teachers—have some type of scandal or crisis in their community. The crises usually involve sex, power, or money, and 90 percent of the scandals are sex related, often with an element of confused power dynamics in *both* the teacher and student.

Sometimes it is worse. Few scandals match the legendary Jonestown and Heaven's Gate mass suicides, but I have been a psychological consultant on a confidential basis to a number of large and small spiritual scandals, and those that involve death make clear how imperative the need is for psychological work on the spiritual path. Often the deaths are an indirect result, or byproduct, of some deep aspect of spiritual bypassing caused by an unrecognized psychological wound in the teacher. It is heartbreaking to see how psychological blindness can co-opt spiritual teachings to result in something as severe as accidental or intentional death.

Even people who do not have a personal relationship to offending spiritual authorities can be rattled by the psychological wounds and blind spots in the teacher and community leadership. They may become uncertain about what is real in the teachings and what is not; they may wonder if they have wasted their time and feel bewildered about which teachings to embrace and which to discard. Spiritual scandals often unearth old traumas in individuals who have not fully healed from their psychological wounds. To address such complexity requires an understanding of *both* the spiritual and psychological dimensions of the circumstance. This recognition further emphasizes how critical it is for everyone in a position of spiritual authority—and anyone who engages in yoga or other spiritual practices—to address their own psychological makeup.

A European teacher once wrote to me seeking psychotherapy, acknowledging that he was using his power to manipulate women into having sex with him. He felt incredibly depressed and anxious about this, and he also felt like a hypocrite as he expounded upon the nondual teachings of yoga and the Hindu teachings of Advaita Vedanta. He wanted to begin therapy, yet he feared that what he might discover about himself would dismantle his identity as a yoga teacher and his organization. Out of this fear (at least to date), he chose not to begin therapy. Sadly, this account is not unusual. I have spoken to other spiritual teachers and their wives, partners, and ex-lovers who also experience this type of struggle within themselves.

However, when people in such circumstances do choose to engage the help of psychotherapy, miraculous things can happen. Although it is often daunting for a teacher to admit to their own errors, face their shame and pride, engage in honest dialogue, and ask for forgiveness from those they have hurt, those teachers who do this work meet unimagined possibilities for healing. Hardened hearts heal, and even people who feel that they have been wronged find a capacity for forgiveness they didn't know they possessed. Often they also discover how they may have unconsciously contributed to the painful dynamic due to their own psychological blindness.

For teachers and students alike, understanding one's own issues is the key. These include self-esteem, relationship to family of origin, how one operates in relationship to a group, what needs were unmet during childhood (and thereby projected onto others), and unresolved traumas. Understanding these issues is crucial if a student is to prevent their own complicity in a spiritual scandal. In this way, psychology enables students to discern which teachers to study with and how to form realistic hopes, thereby reducing the possibility of manipulation and scandal. Hard-won insights also help a student receive optimal benefit because they trust their own process while honoring the skills and gifts of their teachers.

Even teachers without significant mental suffering benefit from psychological self-investigation because it helps them understand the challenges that afflict their students. In a notable example, when the Dalai Lama first came to the West, he encountered prominent self-hatred among Westerners. It took him years to understand what he was encountering and relate to it, as self-hatred was not an aspect of his cultural upbringing.

As I'll talk about more in chapter 6, all of us experience challenges and psychological stumbling blocks simply by virtue of being human. Living at this time, we suffer from particular traumas regardless of whether we are aware of them or think that everything is just fine. I have never encountered a person who has not come across psychological stumbling blocks. If nothing else, we are the recipients of ancestral afflictions that include overlapping challenges pertaining to gender, class, ethnic heritage, immigrations, politics, and our shared environment.

When people engage psychotherapy as a learning experience, rather than something they *have* to do, they are often pleasantly surprised to uncover unconscious forces that dominated their lives. They also enjoy a new capacity to free themselves in ways they had never imagined. By bringing unconscious patterns into the light of awareness, we gain more options, equilibrium, freedom, and even a sense of thriving. People are regularly amazed to discover that self-exploration is not a task to dread, but a joy to uncover. For myself and others, repeating this immersion in the study of our own psyche at each major developmental stage of our lives is invaluable, particularly when we are representatives of spiritual traditions. When undergoing psychotherapy, I often find myself leaping and bounding into sessions, grateful to have a safe, supportive, and effective environment in which the forces of my unconscious can be illuminated. I truly appreciate having a place in which my need to articulate my intensity can be received and held. I plan to engage in therapy at least once a decade in my life, and I encourage my readers to do so as well—not because there is something wrong with us, but because there is something right.

3

WHY PSYCHOLOGY
NEEDS YOGA

The journey of a thousand miles
doesn't begin with the first step.
It begins where you stand.[1]
RAMA JYOTI VERNON

Millions of people worldwide are hooked on yoga—even those who would have least expected to be. Those of us who have tasted its sweet fruits know that there is simply nothing like yoga. It provides detailed maps that describe the vast possibilities of mystical domains of consciousness, much more so than any branch of Western psychology, as well as practical guidance to experientially navigate those domains.

I've been to the banks of the Ganges in Varanasi and Rishikesh, India, multiple times, and I've practiced alongside thousands of others in prayer, asana, meditation, chanting, prostrations, and *pujas* (rituals). I can tell you firsthand that yoga isn't just a philosophy—it's a vibrant, embodied, and living practice.

You don't have to follow Hinduism to benefit from yoga. It's available to anyone who chooses to partake of it. You don't need to be rich, educated, or initiated to enjoy yoga's diverse tapestry of offerings.

YOGA AND CONSCIOUSNESS

In the previous chapter, we explored how Western psychology so brilliantly addresses the contents of the Western psyche, including its trauma and the common afflictions of anxiety, depression, self-esteem, and alienation. In contrast, yoga provides a uniquely detailed and vast body of teachings that address the domain of consciousness itself, specifically describing how transformation takes place within the laboratory of the human mind, body, heart, and spirit.

Yoga—like the religion of Hinduism it's often associated with—entails countless branches, schools, perspectives, texts, approaches, and interpretations due to its thousands of years of development as it moved throughout India, neighboring countries in Asia, and more recently, throughout the world. Although schools of yoga often don't agree with each other in their approach, they share an aim of exploring the mysteries of consciousness. They also address existential questions regarding the nature of awareness, birth and death, the purpose of life, how to live ethically and well, and the deepest possibilities for human awakening.

Yoga addresses participants at whatever level of awareness with which they approach the path. It offers transformational possibilities at various levels of engagement—from those who practice occasionally as a hobby to those for whom the yogic path is the center of their lives. Those who immerse themselves in yoga soon become amazed at how vast and endless the path is. As we dive into the discovery of consciousness as it arises in our own bodies and awareness, we discover that there are endless treasures of knowledge locked away within our minds, bodies, and hearts—for which yoga offers the keys. For myself and countless others, this possibility for self-knowledge is a source of inspiration and great comfort. Engaging yoga wholeheartedly often provides an absolute "okayness" of wherever one finds oneself on the endless journey of self-exploration. As the Tibetan Buddhist master Chögyam Trungpa Rinpoche was fond of saying, "The path is the goal."

Most people enter the path of yoga through posture practice, and for many this is the doorway to yoga's deeper philosophies and more internal practices of breath and meditative awareness. As noted earlier, only three of the 196 aphorisms in the Yoga Sutras refer to asana practice.

The number of ways to engage in yogic discipline is nearly infinite. Other practices include the medical science of Ayurveda; the astrological approach of Jyotish; mantra (sound and chanting); meditative inquiry; visualization; sexuality as a means of discovering realization within the human body; service and devotion; paths that mix with Buddhism and Jainism; and new blends like Om Shalom, Laughter Yoga, and sportive play (like yoga on stand-up paddle boards or wilderness excursions). Whereas some yogic methods aim to transcend the body and our human experience, those I share in this book lend themselves most effectively to blending with psychology and supporting the Western practitioner. Specifically, they aspire to transform our human experience within the body, here on earth, in this lifetime, and in relationship to others.

Yoga is truly vast, concerning itself with the dense areas of con-tracted consciousness as well as the subtlest and most expansive. One of the wonderful qualities of the yogic perspective is that it does not ultimately separate psychological and spiritual well-being. Dr. Marc Halpern, founder of the California College of Ayurveda, writes: "The Ayurvedic understanding of the pathology of disease and the Yogic understanding of the cause of suffering both teach that disease and suffering begin when we forget our true nature as spirit."[2]

Because yoga is so vast, it provides multiple entry points. When practiced under the guidance of a skilled teacher, yoga works with us wherever we are—whether we're healthy or ill, young or old, thin or heavy, flexible or stiff. When I hear people say they can't practice yoga because they're not flexible enough, or they're too fat or too old, my heart aches. I've worked with preschoolers; people who are blind, in wheelchairs, in gangs, addicted to drugs; and even those in the process of dying. Yoga is ultimately an internal practice of awareness and transformation that excludes no one.

A common critique of contemporary yoga is that it has become "dumbed down," meaning that it has strayed from its ancient roots. In fact, I had a young Indian student in one of my trainings who felt quite angry about how yoga, as currently practiced in the Western world, is being "disgraced." This is a certainly a point worth consider-ing, and I have at times—especially as a young practitioner—felt the same way. However, my perspective has softened over time particularly due to a prolonged illness and the influence of wise elders. When I was in my twenties, I interviewed the American Zen Buddhist Roshi Joan Halifax for my book *Halfway Up the Mountain: The Error of Premature Claims to Enlightenment.* I remember lamenting to Roshi about people being careless with spiritual practices and coming across as deluded in their assumptions of their own enlightenment. "Look," she said, "I teach Buddhism to guys on death row where it *really* matters. I don't care what they think about their enlightenment as long as they are practicing something. To me, when people assume premature claims to enlightenment, it's like when we were young girls playing dress-up in our mother's closet. Even if we are just imitating enlightenment, we are somewhere on the path, and that's what counts."

I've contemplated this teaching for years now, and here's how I apply it to this issue: no matter how we approach yoga, it almost always serves us at whatever level we enter the practice. Really, there are as many approaches to the spiritual path as there are individuals. For this reason, teachers and others in positions of authority need to be discerning, psychologically healthy, and committed to continuous learning and growth—not only for their own good, but for the benefit of those who look to them for guidance and support.

YOGA'S INFLUENCE IN THE THERAPY ROOM

When I first opened my psychotherapy practice in my mid-twenties, I tried incredibly hard to "spiritualize" my work. My efforts to add meditation, visualization, or hypnosis sometimes met with success, but mostly they flopped, probably because I was trying too hard. As I furthered my studies over the years, I started to notice that without having to even mention yoga or meditation, my clients just naturally began to express significant spiritual insights. I attribute this to my dedication to my unique spiritual path. I believe that the single variable that determines the likelihood of spiritual insight arising for the client in psychotherapy is the sincerity of practice and spiritual awareness of the therapist themselves. The therapist's own inner work wordlessly transmits an invisible but palpable space into which the client can express their own spiritual and psychological insights and understandings. And when the client experiences their own unfolding wisdom, it is far more powerful than the therapist expressing these ideas overtly or trying to teach them directly. For this reason, I can't emphasize strongly enough the necessity of psychotherapists and yoga teachers to commit themselves to lifelong study, practice, and inner work.

A common critique of conventional psychology and psychotherapy is that they are limited in scope, working primarily with the conditioned mind, personal history, and human behavior. In many cases, this is true. At worst, this shortsightedness manifests as a therapist interpreting a client's longing for God as merely an unfulfilled need from childhood, or viewing a client's relationship with their spiritual teacher only through the lens of dependency or codependency, or interpreting spiritual experiences as delusions or evidence of psychopathology. Often the therapist's or psychiatrist's lack of mirroring of the client's inner experience re-creates the client's early experience of their inner intensity and spiritual essence going unrecognized by their parents and primary caregivers. In order to minimize these pitfalls and allow for the benefits of spiritual insight to unfold, therapists better serve their clients (and themselves) by becoming spiritually informed. At best, the therapeutic process is both psychological and spiritual.

In my Yoga & Psyche trainings, I'm often asked by psychotherapists and mental-health workers how to bring yoga into the therapy room. Chapter 8 covers this in detail, but let's take a look now at some important variables to consider when exploring ways to add yoga to your psychotherapy practice:

1. **Openness of the Client**   When thinking about bringing any specific yogic practices into the therapy room, discuss the idea with clients with an open attitude that allows them to express their own preferences. Present the suggestion as something the client can take or leave, in the present or at some future time. Just because the therapist is passionate about yogic practices and believes they will be useful does not mean the client will

be interested or ready. It's extremely important that the client does not feel that the therapist will be disappointed or that the therapy will be diminished somehow if they opt not to include the proposed practice.

2. **Touch**   When asana practice is included in therapy, physical touch will likely be an important component, even if it's simply helping the client adjust into the postures in an optimal way. It's important to assess the client's openness to touch and explicitly ask permission each and every time, again letting them know it is fine if they prefer that you not touch them. Although physical touch can be tremendously healing, it is often not included in the psychotherapeutic process (in contrast to how touch is used in yoga). Psychotherapy works with the unconscious, and when clients have been physically traumatized or abused in their early lives, they can be understandably sensitive to touch. Keep in mind that several US states also have rules against touch in their licensing process. Even if this is not the case, it is incredibly important that the therapist be sensitive and discerning with respect to any form of physical contact in therapy.

3. **Posture**   For those of us practicing in this new field, there are two distinct ways to approach the use of posture in the therapy room. Amy Weintraub and other colleagues have begun to map specific postures that correlate with supporting clients with particular psychological challenges and ailments. For example, *Baddha Konasana* (Bound Angle Pose, along with other hip openers) may be used to open the client to held emotion around sexuality. *Virabhadrasana* (Warrior Poses I, II, and III) are recommended to help release anger and access power. These are just a couple of examples of many ways asanas, mantras, mudras, and visualizations can be used to work directly with psychological conditions. The other approach, which is particularly useful when the client and therapist are both more experienced in asana, is to tune in to the

client's embodied emotional experience, and encourage and guide them to listen to, and move according to, their body's own inner direction. This process can be guided with or without touch. In my trainings, I encourage participants to explore this second practice with poses they are both averse and attracted to in order to discover and unwind various aspects of their psyches and learn to access the inner wisdom of their own bodies.

4. **Breathing Practices**   Breath practices, or pranayama, are often revelatory for clients. Focusing on the breath brings awareness into the body and connects the mind to it. Pranayama offers an alternative for therapists and clients who want to work with yoga but who are not comfortable using posture and touch. Although more esoteric and complex pranayamas can be helpful in therapy, I have found the simplest practices to be the most accessible and therefore the most effective. For example, the therapist and client can sit with eyes open, facing each other, and the therapist can model breathing fully into the body for three breaths and ask the client to do the practice with them. Or the therapist can teach the client a three-part yogic breath in which the client breathes in first through their lower belly, then into their mid-belly, and then filling their lungs. Then the client exhales first through the lungs, then the upper belly, and then all the way out through the lower belly. To continue, the client pauses and holds their breath for a few seconds, and then repeats the process for two to five more cycles. As I have often told clients, I believe the process of becoming present is as simple as one conscious breath in the body.

5. **Meditation and Visualization**   By learning and exploring mindfulness-based practices themselves, therapists can truly benefit their clients. For example, learning to scan their bodies for areas of tension or numbness in a mindful way introduces clients to somatic awareness, and for many this practice serves as an accessible gateway to getting in touch with their

bodies in a direct way. Visualization practices—such as those that use deities (of any tradition the client resonates with), images of nature, or aspects of ourselves (such as a wiser, more compassionate projection of ourselves that communicates to a more vulnerable or traumatic aspect)—are also helpful in therapy. Again, the therapist does not need to be an expert meditator to bring mindfulness or visualization practices to their clients, but they should be trained, practice regularly, and not teach others techniques that exceed their experience.

6. **Client Feedback**   When I lead trainings, we spend quite a bit of time in mock sessions with new skills, and we also allow ample time for feedback, sharing, and questioning. Sometimes when offering new practices in the therapy or yoga room, we think we must be experts and worry that asking for feedback on a newly introduced technique will result in a lack of trust or respect. In my experience, the opposite is true. When we let our clients know that we are studying new modalities in order to deepen our capacities and that we are open to their feedback about new techniques and exercises, we model vulnerability and receive important information on how best to help the individual client. More importantly, we place them in the position of authority in their own healing process.

   Those of us committed to pioneering this new territory at the intersection of psychology and yoga must be willing to make mistakes—even fall on our faces—and, if we're lucky, laugh at ourselves. Our willingness to be sincere, open, humble, and generous with others and ourselves is a key variable to the successful unfolding of these new innovations.

YOGA AS A COMPLEMENTARY TREATMENT TO PSYCHOLOGICAL WORK

In addition to learning yogic techniques, clients who are pursuing a path of psychological transformation can often find benefit in simultaneously engaging in a regular asana practice or a more intensive immersion in yoga. In my experience, a practice not overly focused on fitness and that doesn't push the practitioner into strenuous poses is particularly complementary to the psychotherapy.

One way that yoga helps in the psychotherapeutic process is to open stuck prana locked within the body. Our psychology is literally contained in the cells of our body. Our wounds and traumas live as contractions, sensations of pain, compromised posture, and physical ailments. Yoga helps to loosen this stuck prana, and helpful psychological practices will work with what is revealed. Yoga further integrates the activated energy and psychological work back into the body. Ideally, a yoga teacher can provide space and instruction to turn the practitioner toward the emotional level of their experience—which is what I teach yoga teachers to do. Yet even when the individual engages the processes of psychological inquiry and yoga asana practice in tandem, they immediately begin to support each other.

One of the gifts of yoga is that it awakens people to the interior life of their bodies. A vast majority of people in the West—and perhaps throughout the world—live their lives with their center of gravity and awareness quite literally their heads. Yoga reveals to people that their bodies are containers of an endless flow of energy. As the body learns to open more, this energy is able to circulate more fluidly.

As I'll explore in chapter 5, when psychotherapy includes an awareness of the body and makes use of embodied awareness in the service of psychological transformation, new possibilities begin to emerge. We learn to be able to digest and process our emotions as sensations in the body as they arise in the moment, and in so doing we find ourselves more at home in our bodies and in our experience. I have found that when teaching somatic approaches to transformation, those who have a background in yoga are often quick to understand and apply this modality. Because they already have access to their bodies at an internal, physical level, yoga practitioners can quickly learn to access and work with the emotional level of their embodied experience.

Trauma-sensitive yoga represents a new approach that draws from trauma theory, attachment theory, neuroscience, and physical yoga in order to treat post-traumatic stress disorder (PTSD) and everyday trauma. The more teachers understand about psychology, somatics, and trauma, the better they can use language that creates psychological safety and offer options to practice that maximize the possibility of healing trauma and minimize re-wounding. In this way, they increase their capacity to serve as true agents of healing.

MEDICATE OR MEDITATE?

When individuals are struggling with more severe symptoms, a synthesis of psychotherapy, yoga, and psychiatry may prove highly effective. Like anything, medication can be used or misused. The argument against psychiatric medication, especially among spiritually oriented people, is that it is too often used to numb experience rather than to support transformation. I have noticed a bias against (not to mention shame about) medication in the yoga and other spiritual communities. People undergoing severe spiritual crises sometimes fear that if they use medication to alleviate some of their acute symptoms, they will somehow miss a chance to pass through the dark night of the soul or lose an opportunity to face their demons once and for all.

My experience working with clients over a long period of time indicates quite the opposite. In his article "Medicate or Meditate?" Buddhist psychiatrist and lifelong meditation practitioner Roger Walsh makes a powerful case for using psychopharmacology in addition to meditation and psychotherapy when treating chronic psychological disorders, even among long-term spiritual practitioners.[3] Although the population cited in Walsh's studies consists of Buddhist practitioners, I believe that the same findings apply to those who practice yoga.

As a psychotherapist, I refer clients to psychiatry when their suffering is either impairing their capacity to function in their daily life or when their psychological pain is so acute that it overwhelms their ability to understand and work toward positive solutions to their challenges. Contrary to common stereotypes, medication does not alleviate the ailments it addresses—there are no pills that bring lasting happiness, neither in psychiatry nor in yoga. Instead, effective medication provides a lever that helps the individual get enough space between themselves and their symptoms to begin to do the necessary inquiry to meet and transform their obstacles.

Psychology also needs yoga to diagnose and treat the very real spiritual processes and crises that people pass through while on the path of yoga—and of spiritual traditions in general. One of my specialties as a psychotherapist has been to work with individuals undergoing spiritual emergence and spiritual emergency—terms coined by psychiatrist Stanislav Grof and his late wife, Christina Grof.

Spiritual emergence refers to an influx of spiritual energy and awareness, such as can occur when individuals first become interested in yoga and meditation and begin to delve into the processes and practices that change their relationships to self and world. This often includes a reevaluation of previous life choices. In the case of *spiritual emergency*, a person becomes flooded with spiritual experiences, insights, and energies that are disruptive and overwhelming. These may cause severe interference or impairment in relationships, work, and daily functioning. Spiritual emergencies can occur spontaneously, as a result of shock or trauma, and sometimes from engaging in intense spiritual practice without the guidance of a skilled teacher.

Spiritual emergencies often arise as a combination of overwhelming spiritual experiences combined with latent tendencies toward psychopathology. When mental-health workers are not versed in spirituality, spiritual openings are usually misdiagnosed and the treatment does not take into account the positive aspects of the experience. This typically results in the client feeling misunderstood. Additionally, this means that the client misses out on the capacities for healing and meaning that spiritual experiences can offer when integrated. A psychotherapist trained in these areas can help the client rebalance and understand their experience in a greater context of overall spiritual development, while simultaneously working directly with the psychological imbalance or psychosis. Meher Baba, a famous Indian mystic, had his closest disciples seek out *masts*, or yogis who were stuck in high states of spiritual experience who had lost the capacity to integrate them. Meher

Baba had these people brought to his ashram where he would personally wash their feet, massage them, and talk with them to help bring them back into their bodies and utilize their spiritual experience in a more embodied, earthly way.

In the case of spiritual emergencies, effective treatment utilizes a skillful combination of traditional and alternative approaches to psychotherapy, alongside a careful consideration of medication with a spiritually informed psychiatrist. Over the years, I have heard countless horror stories of individuals having a profound spiritual experience who were hospitalized, overmedicated, given shock treatment, and misunderstood by their psychiatrists, psychologists, and families. A complementary process of yoga may also be indicated in treatment. However, some spiritual practices can be destabilizing, whereas others may support further balance. A psychotherapist who is also well-trained in yoga can prove invaluable during this time.

The inclusion of "Religious and Spiritual Problems" in the American Psychiatric Association's *Diagnostic and Statistical Manual of Mental Disorders* (DSM) represents a significant breakthrough with respect to the diagnosis and treatment of spiritually oriented psychological challenges. This diagnosis paves the way for various aspects of spiritual crises and emergencies to be taken seriously in psychological and psychiatric treatment. Although psychotherapists, psychiatrists, and mental health-care practitioners trained in yoga are certainly not the norm in their fields, they are increasing in number as yoga gains more acceptance. The Spiritual Emergence Network—a referral source for mental-health practitioners versed in spiritual emergence and emergency throughout the United States—represents another positive step.

As we attempt to traverse the vast domains of consciousness and the gritty crevices of the psyche, passing through the various developmental stages of life and undergoing the inevitable sufferings and traumas that arise within it, the resources that yoga and psychology offer become invaluable allies that help us heal and thrive. I'm convinced that neither tradition alone provides the breadth of maps and tools we need to meet the intensity of the process of being human that both can provide when integrated together.

4

PSYCHOLOGY

A New Western Spirituality

Who looks outside, dreams; who looks inside, awakes.[1]
CARL JUNG

Modern times leave more and more people disillusioned or disenchanted with the traditional forms of religion that they were raised with—if they were raised with religion at all. Yet many people still experience a longing for spiritual direction. When we remember that psychology is a new field that is developing rapidly, as opposed to being something stagnant and fixed, we gain a fresh perspective that examines a spiritual psychology informed by yoga and other spiritual traditions. This chapter proposes that psychology is one of the Western world's significant contributions to contemporary spirituality.

Integrating a depth-psychological approach with the profundity and longevity of the yoga tradition provides us with tools to heal our wounds and make meaning of our experience, while simultaneously encouraging us to discover mystical insights about ourselves and the nature of consciousness. In short, we find out for ourselves, rather than merely following what others teach us to think and feel. My psychotherapy practice is full of spiritually oriented clients who come in with a degree of experience or openness to yoga and other wisdom traditions. Their desire to grow psychologically and spiritually enables us to employ a full range of conventional and innovative approaches to psychotherapy. These include methods with a somatic emphasis in addition to yogic and meditative tools.

At the 2014 International Yoga & Psyche Conference I hosted in San Francisco, 150 visionaries from all over the world presented their own personal research and experience on the intersection of yoga and psychology. (Twelve of these papers are published in *Proceedings of the Yoga & Psyche Conference (2014)*.)[2] One of the keynote presenters, Angela Farmer—an extraordinary "grandmother yogini"—shared that she had personally been integrating depth psychology and yoga for nearly forty years, mostly without access to all the recent innovations in Western psychology. Angela emphasized how fortunate we are to live in a time when all of this new research is at our fingertips, and how precious and imperative it is to take what has become available and build upon it.

NEW MOVEMENTS IN PSYCHOLOGY

The most effective blending of yoga and psychology results when we include traditional, mainstream, and evidence-based approaches to psychology, as well as its newer spiritual developments. Just as our yoga study and practice expand into endless dimensions over a lifetime of immersion, a long-term engagement in a full-spectrum approach to psychology will result in a continuous deepening of our perspective and experience. Before exploring the newer innovations in psychology, it's important to acknowledge that a number of mainstream interventions—specifically, cognitive-oriented ones—are highly effective in managing severe psychological symptoms and crises, namely when it comes to learning effective communication skills and alleviating anxiety, depression, addiction, low self-esteem, and relationship struggles. That being said, let's turn our attention to some of the newer innovations in spiritually oriented psychological approaches.

Transpersonal Psychology

Although the term *transpersonal psychology* was coined and brought into contemporary use by pioneers such as Abraham Maslow, Anthony

Sutich, and Stanislav Grof in the late 1960s, early philosophers and psychologists like William James, Carl Jung, and Roberto Assagioli had been exploring the field since the early 1900s. Today, transpersonal associations exist worldwide, and a small but growing number of undergraduate and graduate programs in transpersonal psychology exist in different countries.

Although much of the early work in the field focused on altered states of consciousness and mystical and meditative experience, modern trends focus on how higher states of consciousness can be integrated and grounded into our daily experience to help us live balanced, meaningful lives while discovering our spiritual possibilities as human beings. Two of my students, Glenn Hartelius and Mary Anne Rardin, and I surveyed forty-one theorists and professors as to how they defined transpersonal psychology more than forty years into its development. We published the results in the *Journal of Transpersonal Psychology* in 2003 and followed up with a synthesis in *The Humanistic Psychologist* in 2007.[3] In short, we found that although there is no common definition of the field, most contemporary theorists concur that a transpersonal approach to psychology addresses a full-spectrum approach to the person. This includes paying attention to wounds, traumas, existing psychopathology, wholeness and thriving, stages of spiritual development, and the challenges and pathologies that can arise in the context of spiritual unfolding. Some of the questions transpersonal psychology asks include:

- How does enduring transformation occur at all levels of a person?

- What constitutes authentic psycho-physical-spiritual integration?

- What are the contexts and practices that cultivate this integration?

Much of the research in the field indicates that mystical experiences alone do not transform people in any lasting way. Transpersonal psychology increasingly focuses on how human beings can draw on psychological and spiritual knowledge and practice to transform in an integrated, embodied manner. It also looks at how such transformation is sustained and further developed into a domain of limitless possibility. Lastly, transpersonal psychology concerns itself with applying personal transformation to various spheres of society, including to politics, education, and environmental concerns.

Transpersonal psychology's examination of how psychopathology and lack of integration can manifest in spiritual development is a valuable contribution to the field. As I mentioned in chapter 2, people immersed in yoga are sometimes prone to fall into gaps of spiritual bypassing. I believe one of the reasons this occurs is because yogic practices enable people to easily experience states of bliss and altered forms of consciousness. However, when not accompanied with psychological inquiry and integration, these states can become so alluring that the practitioner may fall into "traps" of spiritual experience and premature assumptions of enlightenment. These include believing they are more developed than they actually are, dismissing the importance of the messier and more emotional challenges of relationship and communication, endlessly grasping at yogic highs to compensate for human lows, and hoping against odds that enough yoga will heal their psychological wounds and traumas. I cover this subject more thoroughly in one of my early books, *Halfway Up the Mountain: The Error of Premature Claims to Enlightenment.*

Integral Psychology

The field of integral psychology is largely based on the writings and teachings of Sri Aurobindo (introduced in chapter 1). Aurobindo proposed a vision for humanity in which experiences and states of enlightenment are involuted in order to illuminate and transmute all the parts of one's being with the Divine, in addition to transforming society. Other important people who contributed to the evolution of integral psychology include Indra Sen (a close disciple of Aurobindo), Jean Gebser (a Swiss phenomenologist), and Pierre Teilhard de Chardin (a French philosopher and Jesuit priest). More recently, the American philosopher and author Ken Wilber has brought integral theory and integral psychology into wider recognition.

In his All Quadrant/All Level model (AQAL), Wilber suggests that all human knowledge and experience can be diagrammed on a four-quadrant grid, along the axes of "interior-exterior" and "individual-collective."[4] Furthermore, experience can be looked at from at least four perspectives:

1. the individual's subjective sense of self and their own consciousness

2. the person's culture and worldviews

3. the behavioral and physiological aspects of the human experience

4. the social systems and environments that influence our experience[5]

Learning to view their experiences through the lens of these four quadrants has enabled many people to open up a wider perspective with which to understand psychologically and spiritually.

Wilber also suggests that every human being develops according to multiple intelligences or lines. These include cognitive, interpersonal, psychosexual, emotional, and moral lines.[6] I find this distinction particularly relevant here because it addresses how an individual can have profound yogic experiences while continuing to act out sexually, abuse their power and charisma, express weak emotional development, lack appropriate boundaries, and behave unethically.

Mindfulness-Based Approaches

Largely developed by Jon Kabat-Zinn and his colleagues, these widely taught approaches are informed by basic Theravada and Zen meditation, and they're applied to one's psychological conditioning. These approaches include Mindfulness-Based Stress Reduction (MBSR), Mindfulness-Based Cognitive Therapy (MBCT), Dialectical Behavior Therapy (DBT), and Acceptance and Commitment Therapy (ACT). Though they differ in their approaches, each style emphasizes in-the-moment awareness of mental, emotional, and behavioral processes. Their popularity is largely due to a significant and ever-growing body of evidence-based research that demonstrates the effectiveness of their methods. The movement of integrating yoga with psychology emerged after the importation of Buddhism to the West, so the increasing acceptance of Buddhist-based methods into psychology paves important ground for yoga's contribution to the field.

A HERE-AND-NOW PERSPECTIVE ON ONENESS

Connecting with spiritual teachers and sincere practitioners of yoga and other spiritual traditions has changed my perspective on oneness. What I believe in now is softer, less glamorous, and more humble than any ecstatic, continuous "one-with-the-universe" experience of union. My evolving sense of oneness includes a deeper recognition of our shared suffering, as well as an increased sense of responsibility to do our part to express our particular gifts and radiance in the world. As author and activist Joanna Macy has said, "Any awakening worth its grain of salt is going to include all of us."[7]

The most powerful sense of oneness I have ever experienced came at the most unexpected time in my life. It happened when I had been ill for three years with an undiagnosed illness at the same time my heart was shattered by a man I loved deeply. I regularly experienced states of fragmentation, darkness, near-suicidal thoughts, meaninglessness, rage, and total despair. I was due to give a talk at a university but was in such terrible shape that a friend had to drive me to San Francisco from my home outside the city. As we crossed the Golden Gate Bridge, my awareness became drawn to all the people in the city who were psychotic, drug-addicted, violent, suicidal, and broken in countless ways. It dawned on me that I was unequivocally no different from them, and I experienced a deep sense of union with them. Perhaps I wasn't acting out in all the ways that they were, but I was made of the same stuff, and under the right circumstances I was capable of falling into a darkness just as deep as their own. In that whole-bodied recognition, I knew that I had previously imagined myself as somehow different and at least slightly above these people. My work as a psychotherapist has never been the same since that experience. It enabled me to genuinely convey the view that each of us is developing uniquely within the vast context of consciousness, and that we can't objectively evaluate this process other than from the perspective of a whole lifetime. In other words, we are all truly doing the best we can, even if it does not appear that way to others or ourselves. Practitioners and teachers of yoga can easily fall into the trap of feeling subtly superior to those who do not practice and pursue inner knowledge. In this way, their practice of union simultaneously enacts further separation from others.

I have heard my spiritual heroes and mentors speak to this with a more here-and-now, down-to-earth perspective on oneness. I once attended a talk in which a sincere spiritual seeker asked Ram Dass if he still felt that all one needed to do on the spiritual path is "be here now." At the time, Ram Dass was recovering from a life-changing stroke. He paused for a long time and then said softly:

> Yes, I still would say that all we need to do is to "be here
> now," but my understanding of what that means has
> changed over time. I now believe that we must be here now
> with everything—with all parts of ourselves, our emotions,
> our unconscious, all the relationships in our lives, with the
> environmental and political situations that surround us. So
> yes, I do believe we must simply be here now, but we must
> be here with everything and everyone.[8]

Swami Prajnanpad (1891–1974) was an Indian spiritual master and former physics professor who taught Advaita Vedanta in his later years at his ashram in Northern India. As Western disciples began to visit his ashram, Swami Prajnanpad recognized how distinct their psychological makeup was from that of the Indian psyche. He had all of Freud's writings delivered by boat to India. Swami Prajnanpad digested Freud's work and contextualized it within a context of nonduality. He subsequently developed processes and taught his disciples that to be *at one* was to be at one with everything that arose within them, including their full emotional experience. Contrary to other yogic approaches that advocated rising above the messiness of human emotion, personal story, and suffering, Prajnanpad taught his students to unify with these experiences and to learn to relate to them so that they would no longer be overpowered by their emotions.

Arnaud Desjardins, the late Advaita Vedanta master I spoke of in chapter 2, was a disciple of Swami Prajnanpad who taught his students to say *yes* to life. He wasn't just referring to the positive and so-called spiritual aspects of life, but to everything—including anything unpleasant that we would rather not feel. Desjardins also taught that when we find ourselves unable to say yes to whatever arises, we can learn to say yes to the *no*. I help students do this in a direct way through the practice of asana. When guiding them in an embodied and psychological approach to posture practice, I ask students to notice the point of resistance—usually a small voice inside them that says things like "I don't like this pain or strain" or "I should be feeling other than the way I am" or "This shouldn't be here." I then instruct them to try to say yes to this form of their *no* and allow their resistance to just be there, rather than attempting to resist or overpower it. When we are able to do this, a more compassionate psychological space inevitably opens up within us.

After experiencing this subtle shift physically, we can apply it to the everyday aspects of life. We can notice the tension in our bodies at a traffic light when we're running late. We can see when we are frustrated by feeling depressed or anxious and would prefer to experience anything else. At such times, a real-time perspective on oneness and saying yes to the no becomes accessible: we learn to turn toward what we are feeling instead of away from it—not only in our minds but also in our bodies. This seemingly minute shift in our awareness and perspective can often mean the difference between experiencing heaven or hell.

In this way, the yogic teaching of "there is no other" becomes true in the most pragmatic and humble sense of the word, as well as in its transcendent possibility. We begin to recognize that the others we imagine have transcended suffering—or those who we project as having achieved yogic bliss—are just like us. They possess knowledge, wisdom, and gifts in particular areas, and they meet developmental challenges in others. They wrestle with the anxieties of health, aging, and the longing for congruency between their soul's desire and its expression through love, relationships, and work. Although we each express endless and important aspects of diversity, we are also simultaneously part of the same oneness.

PSYCHOLOGY AS AN EXPRESSION OF KARMA

"If somebody had to live my life, why did it have to be me?" quips Buddhist comedian Wes Nisker. When I was a young woman, I felt both intrigued and bothered by the concept of karma. Everyone I knew who remembered their past lives was at some point a princess in Egypt or a medieval European king (and never a village woman in Indonesia or a South American shepherd). It irritated me when people claimed they must have done something terrible in a past life because they were currently suffering—unable to get pregnant, suffering from continuous relationship problems, or getting cancer or a terminal illness. The deeper principles of karma spoke to me, but most of the explanations I heard seemed superficial and overly linear. So I did what any diligent young spiritual student and writer would do—I approached each spiritual teacher or yogi I met on my travels and asked him or her: What is karma?

I resonate with the views of the yogic scholar Robert Svoboda. He says that even the greatest yogis understand but a sliver of the totality of the mystery of karma. Because there is so much misunderstanding of karma, it's valuable to understand that there's much more to it than "payback" as it is generically understood in the Western world. However, the concept didn't become user-friendly and practical to me until I linked it with modern psychology. Doing so has opened up much more self-compassion for how challenging it can be to work through some of our psychological material. In addition, it helped me develop more patience for how long the process of psychological transformation can take, because we are influenced by the "karma" of multigenerational patterns and family lineages, all of which are experienced within our own psychological makeup.

Our personal psychology is how our karmic patterns show up in this lifetime. A general yogic perspective on karma suggests that the individual soul moves through consciousness lifetime after lifetime, incarnating again and again in the school of life in order to complete various tasks and lessons and release contractions of consciousness. The conditions and circumstances of each incarnation are based on forces far vaster and more complicated than most of us can conceive. These forces determine the quality of consciousness we receive, the cultures and families we are born into, the bodies we obtain, and the significant experiences and relationships we encounter. "The accumulated imprints of past lives, rooted in afflictions, will be experienced in present and future lives," writes Patanjali.[9]

Accordingly, if we want to unravel the karma we have accumulated in past lives, we need look no further than our present-life circumstances. Whatever we experience in the present moment is both the fruition of our previous karma and the planting of seeds for future karma. The circumstances we encounter *are* our karma—the expression of our consciousness and the seeds of our future. It is as if we live in an incredible hologram of karma. Our lives reflect the intersection of our family or genealogical karma, the collective karma of our culture, the karma of the earth, and—in some cases—a particular set of karmas expressed through the teachers and communities we encounter on the spiritual journey.

We encounter confrontational moments of bare honesty in life in which we perceive clearly that we are indeed reaping the seeds we have sown. Or maybe we have inherited these seeds through accident, unconsciousness, or misfortune. This most commonly expresses itself in our patterns of intimate relationships and parenting. Although we may try mightily to do otherwise, we tend to enact patterns that were modeled to us, at least until we diligently work to transform them. When people are badly abused as children, whether overtly or subtly, they frequently repeat this abuse in intimate relationships. Perhaps to a lesser degree they repeat these patterns as parents, even when they try to do quite the opposite.

It is possible to trace our current psychological challenges not only to our parents but also to our grandparents, great-grandparents, great-great-grandparents, and even farther back into ancestral time. With close examination, we can discover that so many of the challenges we face are literally passed down through generations as a result of impersonal and unconscious conditioning. Newer methods of group psychological inquiry, such as family-constellation work, endeavor to reveal these multigenerational patterns. We may be shocked to realize that the essence of some of our powerful experiences and strong choices is influenced in an immediate way by ancestors we never even met. These manifest frequently as depression, relationship patterns, illnesses, the age at which we die, and even daily choices we assume are entirely our own (for example, the number of children we have). For many people, it is easier to understand karma when it is framed in this tangible and practical way rather than through a vague notion of the soul moving across lifetimes.

The implications of this are manifold. On the one hand, we are not at fault for the thoughts, feelings, and challenging circumstances that arise in our lives; however, we are at the same time totally responsible for our lives in the present moment and for the implications of our actions. If we can release shame and self-blame while simultaneously strengthening our personal accountability, we can actually transform the damaging patterns that plague our lives and prevent greater joy.

A number of therapies concern themselves with past-life traumas, and spiritual students are endlessly fascinated by who they might have been or what they might have done in their past lifetimes. However, from a practical perspective, we need look no further than our present circumstances. Whether we were a farmer in Mesopotamia, a slave trader in the American South, or a reincarnated yogi is irrelevant for most of us. What is important is whether we are able to meet our present circumstances with a clear and discerning perspective and refrain from acting in such a way that furthers the endless repetition of unfavorable and limiting aspects of our conditioning. From this perspective, psychology becomes a tool we can use to unlock, work with, and evolve our karma.

THE EVOLUTION OF PSYCHOLOGY: AN INVITATION

As compared to yoga—a tradition thousands of years old—psychology is truly nascent in its emergence in the world. Psychology has undergone tremendous growth not only in the past 135 years, but quite recently as major advances continue to emerge. I am not suggesting that it should replace any particular religion or spiritual practice. Rather, I want to emphasize psychology as a truly profound asset to the development of spirituality in the Western world. Neither psychology nor yoga is a fixed development. As discussed earlier, yoga extends into literally infinite possibilities for self-knowledge, whereas psychology has just begun to explore the depths of the psyche. I invite you to consider psychology in its emergence as a powerful contribution to contemporary Western spirituality—perhaps one day becoming a spiritual tradition in and of itself.

PART II

UNWINDING THE PSYCHE THROUGH THE BODY

YOGA, SCIENCE, AND THE BRAIN

coauthored with Gabriel Axel

Measure what is measurable,
and make measurable what is not so.
GALILEO GALILEI[1]

The brain has roughly 100 billion neurons—about the number of stars in the Milky Way galaxy. Each neuron connects to thousands of other neurons, totaling around 150 trillion such connections in the brain. These neuronal connections change continuously, creating new electrochemical circuits with their own magnetic fields that influence the electrical signals of other neurons nearby. The firing of these neurons and the brain's cellular maintenance alone demand 20 percent of the body's resting metabolic energy. The brain—one of the most complex phenomena in the known universe—forms, informs, and conditions our experience of every moment of our lives.

Like yoga, neuroscience concerns itself with the edge that lies between the known and the unknown. Whereas neuroscience focuses on the material constitution of consciousness and uses physical measurement to probe the mind, yoga utilizes introspection to explore the experiential aspects of consciousness and its contents. Like the paths of yoga and other spiritual traditions that predate it, neuroscience poses questions that have existential implications. Accordingly, the field of neuroscience, when approached with curiosity and a sense of wonder, abounds with spiritual potential. Just as yogic and psychotherapeutic frames of mind can transform our self-awareness, neuroscience can similarly illuminate our fundamental nature when we ask the right questions.

YOU CAN CHANGE YOUR BRAIN

The subject of neuroplasticity—the brain's capacity to change or adapt—has gained much public attention in recent years due to its practical relevance: changing our brains can literally change our lives. Neuroplasticity means that our brain is not a fixed entity; instead, the brain is dynamically adaptable—*plastic*—and it changes along with our lived experience. The brain continuously remodels its neural connections in order to optimize our interactions with the world. This occurs chiefly on a biological level by fluctuations in neurotransmission—the transfer of hormones and molecules among neurons. What we call "neuroplasticity" occurs when connections between areas of the brain change and when the density of cells in a particular region of the brain alters.

Yoga and psychology tap in to the brain's neuroplasticity and leverage it for the benefit of the practitioner. Simply put, when we challenge ourselves by stepping outside habitual patterns and direct our mind in some purposeful way, we refine our neural pathways. Yoga utilizes the mind's attention to harmonize various aspects of brain function, and psychology—particularly psychotherapy—guides the mind in a step-by-step manner to question and recontextualize core beliefs, perspectives, and conditioned behaviors.

In yoga, we learn to apply our conscious attention like a blade that cuts through the clutter of the mind. This allows us to attune to information relevant to our goals, and it helps us phase out extraneous information. For example, when a practitioner wishes to place awareness on their breath, they pay attention to signals arising in the body, and the mind becomes more occupied with information about the breath. Research indicates that regular mindful attention changes the density of gray matter in various brain regions, including the insula—an area involved in processing internal bodily signals.[2] We can foster similar changes by engaging in psychotherapy. For example, by paying attention to the way in which certain emotions arise, we can learn to detect and attenuate these emotional signals before they become overwhelming. Additionally, a qualified psychotherapist can help us consider different perspectives and choose new patterns, beliefs, and behaviors accordingly.

Part of our capacity for change is due to neoteny, which literally means "to extend the new." Neoteny describes the tendency of organisms to retain youthful features into adulthood. In human characteristics, we see neoteny such as relatively round skulls, flattened faces, and small teeth—and humans retain these features into adulthood to a greater degree than most other primates. But the epitome of neoteny in humans is the fact that we retain a larger window of neuroplasticity than other primates during development. Specifically, particular genes involved in our neural development remain active far longer than those of other primates.[3] Over the course of our development from childhood to adulthood, our brain evolves like a symphony of structural changes set off by cascades of genetic signals.[4] This expanded window of neuroplasticity means that we are vulnerable to change, but we are simultaneously capable of adapting to it. We can take advantage of this evolutionary feature of our basic makeup through the various methods presented by yoga and psychology.

HOW NEUROSCIENCE CAN EMPOWER YOGA AND PSYCHOLOGY

Humans tend to interpret living systems according to the prevailing needs and belief systems of the times in which they live. Currently, we find ourselves in an era that prioritizes concreteness, so we emphasize the material constituents and mechanisms of life. From this approach, neuroscientists have made tremendous advances over the past few decades, and they are now able to describe the links between specific psychological functions and the activity in particular brain regions.

For example, research in recent years has shed light on a malleable network of brain connections, called the default mode network (DMN), which is largely responsible for generating our sense of selfhood.[5] Neuroscience examines the biological mechanisms that shape experience, "popping the hood" on the engine of our brains and allowing us to map with anatomical accuracy the layers of our being. With novel research tools, models, and treatments, neuroscience is on the cutting edge of self-understanding and mind-body science.

Psychology and yoga can inform the endeavors of neuroscience by offering tools for navigating, regulating, and making sense of our lived experience. Psychology (especially psychotherapy) addresses the process of understanding ourselves by helping us to deconstruct and reconstruct our experience. Yoga, on the other hand, aims to bring coherence to our experience—the unification of different strands of our being. To the integration of these fields, neuroscience brings precision in four important ways: measurability, referentiality, direct access, and co-evolution.

1. **Measurability**   By anchoring felt experience in objective structures, we ground the seemingly ineffable experiences we have in yoga and psychology into more concrete language. Making precise measurements affords researchers and practitioners the ability to collect data, compare results, and draw conclusions based on that data. Measurability allows for the potential benefits of yoga and psychology to be quantified. We can, for example, now measure the effects of meditation and psychotherapy on changes in brain regions that regulate how we process emotions.[6] This allows for comparisons among different practices and groups of people, as well as positively changing protocols in clinical medicine, preventive health, yoga instruction, and elsewhere.

2. **Referentiality**   Understanding the nuts and bolts of the nervous system gives us reference points—objective anchors of meaning—for the practice of yoga and psychology. It is easy to underestimate how much the language we use affects

how we perceive our condition and the world in which we find ourselves. The mind isn't some kind of passive sponge. It actively seeks out data to construct and inform its worldview, and neuroscience offers increasingly precise information that serves to enrich our interpretations of our experience and the world around us. By studying and interpreting yogic techniques and psychotherapeutic methods, neuroscience helps us understand our internal workings and develop new metaphors with which to anchor our experiences, thereby empowering and enlivening practice in a robust, empirical, and meaningful way.

3. **Direct access**   The latest brain models suggest that our subjective experience is a form of virtual reality hosted by the nervous system. There is a continuity—not a chasm—between our physical neurons and the quality and contents of our subjective experience. This means that subjective experience is literally a window into our neurobiology. There is no aspect of our experience that is not in some manner represented in our neurobiology; similarly, every aspect of our experience is conditioned by our underlying neurobiology. Neuroscience asserts that the nervous system produces subjective experience as a simplified schema of its own complex neural activity. By polishing our lens through yoga and psychology, our felt experience shows us precisely the information we need to direct our actions in the world as we choose.

The fundamental potential of neuroplasticity arises from the fact that there is a continuity between our felt experience and the nervous system. Accordingly, if we want to change our brain, we must change our experience, and we must do so by finding ways to manipulate experiences that alter our underlying neurobiology—as above, so below. We need tools that empower us to better link the subjective and objective dimensions of our being, and both yoga and psychology support us toward this end.

4. **Co-evolution** Yoga, psychology, and neuroscience are all complementary and capable of informing each other in ways that optimize the possibility for integral self-understanding. Yoga is not a static gift from antiquity; it is an ever-evolving art form influenced by every practitioner. The same holds true for the younger, but rapidly evolving, field of Western psychology. By bringing neuroscience into the mix, we can contribute to the further development of each of these fields as well as to their integration. In this way, we can recombine and repurpose techniques for personal needs and support transformation in a changing world.

Our complex world presents unique challenges that were nonexistent in previous historical eras when various philosophies of yoga and the originating approaches to psychotherapy were developed. Yoga and psychology must be efficacious for the individual who employs them. The precision of neuroscience grants myriad opportunities for designing still more effective and relevant processes and practices tailored to the needs and dispositions of individuals.

HOW YOGA AND THERAPY HELP CALM US

Over the years, scientists have been working on ways to demonstrate how yoga and psychology positively affect the nervous system, thereby contributing to our health and well-being. One helpful method developed by Stephen Porges, PhD, is called Polyvagal Theory, which is used to describe the value of yoga from a neurological perspective.[7] This theory elucidates how the nervous system adapts to its environment and how this adaptation interplays with psychological experience. Polyvagal Theory is relevant for understanding a range of processes found in psychology and yoga—for example: a client learning techniques to regulate their emotions in therapy, or a yoga practitioner consciously managing their breath or heart rate.

Polyvagal Theory focuses on the activities of the vagus nerve, which descends from the base of the brain down through the internal organs

of the body. The vagus nerve controls various functions of the autonomic nervous system (ANS)—a branch of the nervous system that
regulates unconscious actions such as heart rate, respiration, digestion,
pupillary response, and sexual arousal. Specifically, the vagus nerve
conducts parasympathetic activities for the ANS, meaning it supports
activities related to rest and digestion.

Polyvagal Theory specifies two pathways of the vagus nerve. One
is an evolutionarily older tract (distinctive of reptiles) associated with
the immobilization response an animal experiences when faced with a
life-threatening circumstance. The other pathway is a result of a later
development in mammals that prioritizes social bonding by damp-
ening sympathetic fight-or-flight behaviors. This results in decreased
fear in response to a threatening situation. This latter vagal pathway
allows us to become more sensitive to our immediate surroundings
and enables us to respond to changes from a mature, adult perspective rather than to remain stuck in older, more conditioned responses.
The more adaptive mammalian vagal pathway became integrated with
parts of the brain stem that regulate muscle control of facial expression,
eye gaze, and speech. All of these relate to the connection between
bodily states and how we express ourselves socially.

Vagus nerve activity—or vagal tone—is typically measured by heart
rate variability (HRV) during the breath cycle. The breath naturally
modulates vagal tone: during inhalation the heart rate increases; during
exhalation it decreases. In experienced practitioners of yoga and meditation, HRV, and thus vagal tone, increases. This results in an improved
capacity to regulate your nervous system, thereby reducing erratic and
emotional responses and bringing about greater calm, ease, and overall
well-being.[8] In turn, this capacity enables us to move out of negative
states and patterns, and it also allows us access to healthier and more pro-
ductive choices. One unique study utilizing brain imaging demonstrated
that experienced meditators have an increased density of grey matter in
regions of the brain stem that control heart rate and respiration.[9]

A variety of physical and mental benefits are associated with
increased vagal tone, which has been shown to decrease with aging,
obesity, and cardiovascular disease.[10] It is also positively associated

with more efficient gas exchange in the lungs.[11] This has implications for the yogic breathing practices of pranayama, which may enhance gas exchange and thereby regulate physiological functioning in desired ways. More research is needed in this area, however, in order to elucidate the connection between vagal tone and various forms of pranayama. On an emotional level, higher vagal tone in adolescents has been associated with increased empathy and a healthy attachment with their mothers,[12] whereas lower vagal tone has been associated with various psychiatric disorders, impulsivity, and difficulty regulating emotions.[13] Positive emotions have also been shown to increase vagal tone, which in turn further encourages positive emotions.[14]

When we mindfully hold a yoga posture or consciously regulate our emotions, our vagal tone influences our felt experience. When we shift our attention from the busy external world and pay attention to internal functions such as our breath, heartbeat, and internal experience, this shift automatically enhances vagal functioning. This brings us greater health and well-being, and it allows us to become more attuned with ourselves and others.

Over the course of evolution, the pathway of the vagus nerve has wonderfully shifted from one tuned for fear response to one focused on social bonding and empathy. Increased vagal tone, brought about through yogic and psychotherapeutic processes, acts as a kind of lubricant for the nervous system, whereby our healthier human capacities are promoted and given more bandwidth. As we explore how the brain and nervous system work while we're in a yoga posture, we can keep in mind the wonders of the vagus nerve in helping us synergize our mind and body.

TOURING THE NERVOUS SYSTEM THROUGH YOGA

For the sake of simplification, let's look at six major levels of the nervous system: the raw senses, autonomic function and coordination, emotion, cognition, metacognition, and self-sense. These levels extend out from the central neural axis that runs from the spinal cord up through the brain, and they layer on top of each other like a pyramid that hierarchically progresses from the most primitive functions to the most complex. Whereas the nervous system is often described in an objective and traditionally scientific manner, we can turn this otherwise technical information into practical knowledge by applying it to yoga practice.

Let's look at these layers through the lens of Tree Pose, or *Vrksasana* in Sanskrit. I suggest reading this section one time through and then actually following the instructions in a subsequent read. That being said, to assume this asana, you balance on one leg with the other foot pressed into the thigh or calf of the standing leg. This pose benefits balance, focus, and concentration; it also strengthens the ankles and knees. As you inhabit Tree Pose, pay attention to the functions afforded by each layer of the nervous system. Doing so will reveal different aspects of your practice to refine and re-integrate, resulting in a practice that truly brings your nervous system to life.

1. **The Raw Senses** While you are positioned in Tree Pose, what information is available to you? At the bottom layer are the *exteroceptive* senses that perceive the external world (touch, smell, sight, taste, and hearing). Next are the *proprioceptive* senses—those that perceive the positions of neighboring body parts relative to each other. Also at play is the *equilibrioceptive* sense, which measures the position of the body relative to gravity. As you might guess, these latter two categories are quite important in yoga.

   In Tree Pose, your proprioception detects that one leg is bent at the knee and the other leg is straight. Proprioceptive input from various body parts tells us where the body is in space, which allows us to make adjustments to our limbs in real time. In contrast, equilibrioception influences how we calibrate balance in the pose from moment to moment, which develops improved balance over time. We sense balance via movements of a fluid in the inner ear that translate into neural signals. Equilibrioception plays a major role in anchoring consciousness in the physical body,[15] and Tree Pose instills a sense of grounding and stillness as we stabilize our balance.

2. **Autonomic Function and Coordination**   Can you sense your heartbeat and breath while in Tree Pose? You cultivate the stability discovered through equilibrioception through autonomic functions controlled by the medulla and pons in the brain stem. As discussed earlier in this chapter, autonomic function refers to the regulation of ordinarily unconscious processes in the body like heartbeat or breath. These processes are associated with *interoception*—the detection of internal bodily signals. Concentrating attention on particular bodily signals—an ability that yoga, somatics, and other mind-body practices have been scientifically demonstrated to improve—can consciously regulate interoception.[16] Directing and holding your attention on internal states increases neural activity in the insula, a region in the brain crucial to interoception.[17] With practice, breathing becomes smoother, heart rate slows, and the mind relaxes and becomes more still.

While in this pose, you might be shaky and vibrating or steady and stable. The cerebellum, also at the base of the brain, coordinates the timing of all sensory and motor signals in order to create a fluid experience. Over time, this results in smoother and more integrated movements. By coordinating the breath and movements in a synchronous manner, repeated practice of yoga improves steadiness and equilibrium.

3. **Emotion**   What is your emotional experience while in Tree Pose? Do any fears or past traumas influence your current experience, even unconsciously? The limbic system—comprised of numerous brain regions above the brain stem—is associated with assigning emotional value to experience. The amygdala is the part of the limbic system associated with negative or fear-based emotions; it is activity in the amygdala that turns emotional experience into reactivity. Traumatic experiences sensitize activity in the amygdala, which can make us get stuck in survival mode if left unchecked.[18]

Strong emotions and unhealed wounds can arise when practicing yoga. When they do come up, teachers and practitioners who are psychologically informed have an opportunity to process traumas that they might have held within them for a lifetime. As a yogi's practice matures, the amygdala's response to negative emotional stimuli is dampened.[19] This results in decreased fear and reactivity, which means an increased ability to process whatever emotional content arises in practice.

4. **Cognition**   Various thoughts arise in different levels of awareness from moment to moment. These thoughts are the responsibility of a large part of the cortex and its outermost layer, the neocortex—both layered above the major structures of the limbic system. The cortex and neocortex play a key role in our decision-making, judgments, and the language we use, among other things.

These cognitive processes have the potential to guide our experience in a useful way. They can also work to our detriment in the form of negative self-talk, unfavorable comparisons, self-negation, and other psychological ailments so common among yoga practitioners in the West. (One example would be judging oneself as lacking the flexibility of other practitioners in yoga class.) Discursive thought and self-talk are inevitable, of course, and cognitive capacities enable us to assess our levels of pain or discomfort. Cognition also allows us to investigate subtle and otherwise hidden issues like the expectations and projections we bring to our practice, or our attempts to suppress emotional pain and trauma through physical exertion.

Incoming sensory and emotional tributaries from the lower layers of the neural hierarchy merge into a cogent stream of information. This multisensory integration primarily occurs in the cortex and neocortex. When we inhabit an asana like Tree Pose with ease and stability, we experience multisensory integration in a refined and cohesive way. Mindfully paying attention to the body as we practice harnesses neuroplasticity, which refines the neural pathways associated with processing signals from the body.

5. **Metacognition**   Once we gain familiarity and comfort in Tree Pose and other asanas, the possibilities truly begin to open up. Metacognition—the "thinking about thinking" function that resides in the more abstract layers farther up the nervous-system hierarchy—is often referred to as an executive function because it exerts control over a number of the brain's other functions. Generally, metacognition includes problem-solving, self-monitoring, and volition. These functions are governed in large part by the frontal lobe of the brain, which includes subregions of the prefrontal cortex (PFC) in concert with other brain regions. Metacognition is an extension of some of the previous cognitive functions, such as judgment and decision-making, and it affords us the capacity to become increasingly aware of our emotional and cognitive patterns. In practical terms, once we recognize that we have attained equilibrium in one part of a posture, metacognition allows us to consider the next level of development in a given pose or our overall practice.

Significantly, metacognition helps us become cognizant of factors that influence our performance and learning process, thereby creating the opportunity for change. Using higher goals to will us through a difficult experience—for example, sustaining a pose that elicits unpleasant emotions in order to process and integrate them—relies in part on metacognition. Similarly, when we set an intention at the beginning of a yogic or meditative practice, or within a psychotherapy session, and we carry it forth effectively, we engage our metacognitive capabilities.

Metacognition helps us observe our behavior and compare it to our desired goals and intentions. In this way, we can align our practice with all aspects of our daily lives in order to bring us closer to the life we most deeply yearn for. Metacognition allows us to greet ever-changing circumstances with optimal responsiveness, which is one of the tremendous gifts of yoga, psychology, and similarly transformative practices.

6. **Self-Sense**   What does it feel like to be *you* while in Tree Pose? The self-sense is the most abstract layer of the nervous-system hierarchy; it's associated with the brain's DMN (default mode network). The self-sense is the process in which the nervous system actively binds together neural information into a coherent, subjective experience. It is the part of the nervous system that generates a sense of selfhood, and it is also the capacity that allows the feeling of being *me* to occur. The self-sense is like magic glue that coheres the various aspects of yourself to produce the impression of having a unified self and possessing a particular identity. Through informed and dedicated yoga practice, in addition to dynamic psychological inquiry, we can develop a healthy self-sense.

The DMN is active when the mind is idle. It's also at work during daydreaming and self-reflection. The DMN gets its name because it is characteristically our default mode of mental activity. It's associated with regions that run along the midline of the brain, such as the medial prefrontal cortex (mPFC) and other regions in the neocortex, including the angular gyrus (AG) and temporoparietal junction (TPJ). Together, these areas of the brain regulate the processing of the sense of control over our actions, as well as self-consciousness.[20]

Our self-sense is the distilled product of all nervous system activity. Even without our knowing it, the self-sense contains the information necessary for us to live and interact with others. The final indicator of the quality of our experience in Tree Pose or other yogic practices is how it affects our sense of self. There are aspects of yogic and psychological experience that further explore the self-sense in relationship to mystical and nondual states of awareness. These esoteric aspects of yogic and meditative practice are not addressed with much depth in this book, but neuroscience and psychology are increasingly exploring these exciting areas.

⁂

As you can see, the practitioner in Tree Pose (or any pose, of course) experiences the different layers of neural processing stacked atop each other, even if unconsciously. The structure and experience of Tree Pose itself reflect the hierarchical structure of the nervous system; the stability of the lower, sensory layers is like the trunk of a tree, whereas the higher, abstract layers are like the tree's branches.

Neuroscience offers new insight into why people of different cultures, ages, and degrees of physical health consistently experience the benefits of yoga practice. An approach to yoga that is informed by neuroscience uses new and helpful reference points to inform our felt experience in all aspects of our practice. This model can be used to explore different asanas and can be applied to our yoga practice or experience of psychotherapy.

MINDFULNESS RESEARCH: STAGES IN THE YOGIC JOURNEY

Due in part to the surge in interest in Buddhist-based mindfulness practices and the studies on their benefits, most of the new neuroscientific research has to do with meditation. Admittedly, it's also more difficult to scan the brain of someone moving, as is often the case with asana practice, than someone sitting still. However, the research is applicable in principle to the practice of yoga because the tradition embraces practices, including meditation, that do not involve movement—and movement can be performed mindfully.

Regardless of whether the practice includes movement or not, a person engaged in meditation goes through four cognitive phases that tend to cycle repetitively as they progress toward concentration.[21] Let's look at each of these four phases in more detail.

Phase 1 *Mind wandering* is associated with the DMN—areas of the brain that are active when the mind is in its default state of rest. In this phase, the mind seems cluttered with thoughts and feelings all scrambling to be at the center of attention. The meditator may remain distracted by what seems like an endless barrage for some period of time. The brain remains in this state especially when it is not engaged in a specific task.

Phase 2 *Becoming aware of mind wandering* occurs when we mobilize a conscious mind-body practice. This phase involves purposefully placing our attention in order to steer our practice, and this effort reveals itself as activation in the insula. As noted previously, the insula is characteristic of interoceptive awareness and self-awareness. In this way, cognizance of the mind's habitual wandering is a form of metacognition—thinking about thinking—that sets the stage for neuroplasticity. Just to arrive at this stage of meditation is quite an accomplishment, as most people never cultivate any sustained awareness of how their mind meanders from one topic to the next. Practitioners should recognize the value of this second phase, because it can take years to arrive here with any regularity. Without knowing this, beginners often become discouraged.

Phase 3 *Shifting out of wandering* is like flexing a muscle or changing gears in a car. This phase involves the executive function of the brain, recruiting regions like the dorsolateral prefrontal cortex (dlPFC) and the posterior parietal cortex. The practitioner arrives at this phase through consciously and consistently bringing their attention out of unfocused wandering. Much like training a muscle, we go through high and low points of practice, and—as in the previous stage—it is easy to feel discouraged. Unfortunately, meditators can judge themselves harshly at this stage, lose interest, or give up entirely if they do not recognize just how important this phase is in training the neural muscles of concentration.

Phase 4 *Focusing*, the fourth phase, means that the practitioner has gained some meditative stability and can remain for some time in a concentrative state. This achievement shows up as sustained activation in the dlPFC. At this phase, progressive layers of our mind reveal themselves—both within a practice session and "off the cushion" over time. When the mind eventually starts to wander again, the cycle begins anew, and the practitioner passes through the phases once more to regain focus. With practice, the amount of effort, time, and repetition it takes to go through the cycles decreases, with less time occupied in the earlier phases and more time spent in a focused state.

The progression described here is dynamic and not necessarily linear. Our practice and spiritual growth ebb and flow with life's organic rhythms, and the challenging aspects of life (aging, disease, grief, and so on) will naturally affect one's experience of practice, as well as one's progress.

That being said, as a practitioner traverses through the phases from a default mode of mind wandering to a focused state, there are certain neural signatures that represent this transition over the long term.[22] For those who have not practiced as much, most of their work lies in initiating the movement of the mind toward focus. This effort shows up as increased activity in the medial prefrontal cortex, which is the part of the prefrontal cortex that lies along the brain's midline and is part of the default mode network. In contrast, more experienced meditators tend to show less use of the medial prefrontal cortex and instead exhibit a different set of neural connections that represent more brain resources allotted to maintaining the states of focus.[23] Even when shifting away from mind wandering and into a focused state, more experienced practitioners show less activity in the medial prefrontal cortex.[24] Maintaining focus over time is associated with an increased role of the striatum, a midbrain structure involved in optimal control of behavior.[25]

Experienced meditators show an increased ability to sustain deeper meditative states and don't have to work so hard to get there. When beginners learn to drive a car, their movements are jerky—there may be more accelerating and decelerating, as if they're constantly in stop-and-go traffic. More experienced drivers, however, drive more smoothly and efficiently, and it's the same with meditation. With consistent practice, practitioners cultivate neural pathways that are competent and advantageous, thus allowing them to maintain deeper states of concentration in their practice.

COMPONENTS OF MIND-BODY PRACTICE

When we truly engage in mind-body practices—or follow any transformative path, really—we can sometimes feel as if we're groping our way around in the dark, uncharted territory of the mind. Any sincere practitioner will inevitably encounter uncertainty and doubt. For this reason, we can rely on experts and teachers to help us through, and we can also look for some empirically grounded guideposts. This section covers four such guideposts—essential components, actually—that have been articulated by research, namely studies in neuroscience that look at different types of practice across various spiritual traditions and levels of meditative proficiency.[26] Understanding these key components of mind-body practice can help us understand how neuroscience accounts for the some of the profound changes we experience in both yoga and psychotherapy. These guideposts also orient us through the sometimes baffling terrain of the mind and teach us a shared language to aid in communicating our experiences.

Attention The basic platform upon which any mind-body practice operates is attention. Meditation involves, first and foremost, a fine-tuning of attention. Attention represents the precision—the efficient attunement—of neural connections and networks in processing information. When we pay attention through practice, we fine-tune the connections in the brain involved in that specific experience, so attention is the mechanism that enables neuroplasticity. As we practice remaining attentive to the breath or to a particular bodily sensation in yoga or meditation, we strengthen the neural pathways involved in their detection, and we thereby become more sensitive to such signals as they arise in the future.

As we explored earlier, the prefrontal cortex (along with other areas in the brain) controls where conscious attention goes. Studies comparing novice and advanced meditators have shown that long-term practice changes the part of the prefrontal cortex that is predominant during attention in meditation.[27] In the early stages of practice, the medial prefrontal cortex—a part of the default mode network implicated in mind wandering—is primarily active as we learn to train the mind to note incompatible, distracting, and intrusive thoughts. In later stages of practice, the dorsolateral prefrontal cortex takes over to sustain vigilant attention over experience as it arises. This transition results in less overt effort, and a sense of effortless attentiveness to experience as it naturally arises.

Emotion Regulation   Another important component of mind-body neuroscience is emotion regulation. As discussed before, emotions are generally associated with the limbic system. Even in the most rational of minds, emotions impart bias on the brain's cognitive operations, resulting in thoughts that are often rationalizations of unconscious signals from the body.[28] Emotion regulation requires learning to reassess our belief systems and reprogram our responses to events or people that might normally trigger us. In other words, we take a step back and learn to evaluate our interpretations of experience from other perspectives.

Neuroscience shows us that the prefrontal cortex mitigates activity in the amygdala, the region associated with fear that tends to skew our perception.[29] Over time, those engaging in mind-body practice use less effort to regulate their emotions by way of reassessing their experience. Instead, they become more capable of being mindfully present with feelings as they arise. This means that they are better able to allow sensations to arise in the body and mind, moment to moment, with less emotional resistance.

Self-induced regulation through mind-body practice can also occur with the guidance of a psychotherapist who is emotionally attuned to the practitioner. One study illustrates that a client's brain was activated in a similar manner, whether their emotions were regulated by themselves or a skilled psychotherapist.[30] This finding points to the power of the connection between psychology and yoga (as well as other mind-body methods), and illustrates that consciously interacting with others can elicit profound psychological shifts in us.

Self-Awareness   A well-known result of yoga and other mind-body practices that attracts many practitioners is self-awareness. Sustained mind-body practice can modify and upgrade the way the nervous system processes self-awareness. For example, long-term practice enables us to erode an egocentric perspective, evolve our self-awareness, and become more integrated with the world around us. Through various forms of conditioning, we can feel as if we are separate from the world, but as our attention becomes more refined—represented by enhanced connectivity between the dorsolateral prefrontal cortex and the default mode network—we gain a sense of continuity (i.e., nonseparation) between the self and its environment.[31] Additionally, the default mode network (and therefore the self-sense) becomes more connected with limbic regions that bring about increased connection with the body.[32]

Intention   A high-level function regulated by the brain's executive network, intention involves creating a goal to contextualize practice.[33] In the context of yoga, intentionality aids attention in the process of neuroplasticity, acting like a compass to direct our practice toward the achievement of desired goals. Intentions can include devotion, nonattachment, compassion, forgiveness, love, or simply improved health. Intention ultimately connects and drives the other components (attention, emotional regulation, and self-awareness), sculpting the dynamic architecture of the brain.

NERVOUS SYSTEM ARCHITECTURE: REMODELING YOUR BRAIN

The brain has an elegant way of computing information. What we call *top-down* streams refers to the higher layers of the nervous system that influence the lower layers, whereas *bottom-up* streams refer to the influence of incoming sensory information on the higher layers of the brain's hierarchy. In the early stages of practice, we exert top-down control on the mind and body as we attempt to make positive changes. After this corrective phase, and as we become more proficient in our yogic or psychological practice, the brain begins to progressively process information in a more bottom-up mode. This transition represents our growing capacity to meet our immediate experience with more clarity and objectivity.[34]

Top-down and bottom-up streams interact at all levels of the nervous-system hierarchy at all times. The brain has a particular scheme for dealing with the interaction of these streams of information known as predictive processing—the brain creates a model of the world in an attempt to increase a sense of predictability and certainty in an uncertain environment. Through yogic and psychological practices, we can update the model of the world fabricated by the nervous system and essentially "remodel" our brains.

The brain pulls information from past experience to generate expectations and predictions about present circumstances, and these directly influence our perception. This process works something like a double-edged sword, however, in that our nervous system produces both adaptive and maladaptive responses and habits. For instance, a child who touches a hot stove and experiences the ensuing pain will learn to not repeat that behavior. This is a positive, adaptive response. On the other hand, some of the brain's conditioned responses are outdated in that they are based on past experience that is no longer occurring. For example, in addition to avoiding the hot stove, the child suffers a fear response every time they get near a stove, whether or not it is lit. Ideally, psychotherapy helps clients uncover unconscious perceptions, patterns, and actions they enact in the present that are based on maladaptive and often forgotten perceptions from the past. In this way, effective psychotherapy helps clients enact more positive and healthy responses to past programming.

Yoga and psychology leverage the brain's malleability, using the principle of neuroplasticity to update the brain's model of the world. As we move through life, we inevitably get stuck in habitual loops of unhelpful behaviors and belief systems that hinder our well-being. When we attempt to transform negative patterns into more positive ones through yoga, psychotherapy, or other transformational disciplines, we can initially experience a type of friction with the world. Our old, conditioned habits appear to conflict with our new goals, or we may encounter fears about change or engaging the unknown, even if we know we are moving in a positive direction. This occurs because the old neural patterns are still at play. When we intentionally try to create healthy patterns and beliefs, the upper cognitive layers transmit signals in a top-down direction through the rest of the nervous system, resulting in an attempt to make new predictions or develop new expectations about how we perceive the world. This process conflicts with ingrained behaviors and expectations. This initial incongruence between top-down and bottom-up streams of information is a normal part of intention-based transformative practices.

As the predictive processing architecture of our brain naturally attempts to create a model of the world that copes with uncertainty, we invariably bump up against information that conflicts with its expectations. *Prediction error* refers to the way our nervous system registers the discrepancy between our new intention-based top-down predictions and our habitually encountered bottom-up patterns of sensory information. The brain deals with this either by acting out a conditioned response or by enacting a new, updated response.

In the first approach, when we encounter a contradiction between what we expect and what we perceive, the brain selectively filters the input we receive from the world to confirm what we already believe. For example, if during yoga practice we encounter a difficult emotional experience, we might have a knee-jerk avoidance response in which we recoil from the experience and move into a more comfortable emotion or thought. In this scenario, no substantial upgrade or intention-based neural remodeling occurs. This is precisely how we get stuck in habits and stagnate growth, thereby unwittingly limiting our transformative process.

On the other hand, when we persevere through the difficulties of yogic and psychological practice, the nervous system rewires old beliefs and behaviors. In this scenario, when we encounter a difficult emotion during yoga practice, instead of avoiding it we choose to remain present, learn to understand and process through it with effective psychotherapeutic tools, and thus change our perspective about it. This skillful persistence results in a harmonious reconciliation of prediction error, or discrepancy, between the new, intention-driven expectations that arise through practice and our conditioned, habituated ways of interacting with the world. In this way, top-down efforts pay off by tuning our attention, regulating emotions, and changing self-awareness. Additionally, top-down control gradually gives way to greater acceptance of bottom-up information as it arises. For this reason, we need long-term, sustained efforts in both psychological and yogic practices to create lasting changes. We consciously remodel our brains by moving against the neural "grooves" that have been operant throughout our lives.

It is important to understand that our nervous system, by default, places more weight on past experience than on new, intention-driven experience. It also generally puts more attention on negative emotions and thoughts than on positive ones. Neuroscience refers to this as the *negativity bias*.[35] Our brains evolved to respond quickly to threats to our survival in a harsh and unpredictable world. Therefore, setting intentions for mindfully venturing into unfamiliar territory—even when moving toward healthy, adaptive responses—is something of an uphill battle. Even when we embrace positive, life-affirming beliefs and behaviors, it may feel challenging, uncomfortable, and even wrong because our conditioned survival response is threatened.

Predictive processing offers a broad lens through which we can understand how the nervous system computes our conscious efforts—both within a given yoga or psychotherapy session, as well as through long-term practice. In modern life, we are fortunate to have access to both the ancient teachings of yoga and the modern developments in psychology discussed throughout this book, but we also can rely on the contributions of neuroscience that demonstrate to us that we can change our lives through changing our brains. More to the point, we are able to integrate the unifying intention of yoga, the step-by-step process of psychology, and neuroplasticity to remodel our brains. Rather than blindly accepting the brain's outdated models of the world, we can cultivate a world of our own making. For those who engage life itself as a transformational path, there is no end to this remodeling because we can always refine the architecture of our nervous system.

NEW HORIZONS: UNITING SCIENCE AND YOGA FOR A BRIGHTER FUTURE

By applying the growing body of knowledge regarding the interaction of yoga and psychology with the nervous system, a plethora of opportunities will continue to arise to enhance the merger of these highly complementary fields. The following areas represent new frontiers of research and development in the connection among the three:

Transformative neurotechnology We can develop more specific technologies—for example, transcranial direct-current stimulation (tDCS) and transcranial pulsed ultrasound (TPU)—to stimulate the brain in order to enhance its function. We can modulate brain activity with technology to facilitate desired states of consciousness (such as meditative focus) and develop new ways of understanding and connecting with the body. Additionally, we can enhance psychological processes and access subtle domains of consciousness. The use of virtual reality will hopefully grow into a powerful tool that guides participants into altered states of consciousness and promotes positive change. Neurotechnology has the potential to draw people from a wide variety of disciplines who might not otherwise be attracted to yogic or psychological insights and practices.

Subtle functions Neuroscientific studies of the physical body as it relates to yoga and psychology are well underway and will inevitably continue to increase at a rapid pace. What remains largely unexplored is the neuroscience of subtler aspects such as the yogic domains of prana, *nadis*, *chakras*, *kundalini*, and *tantra*, as well as transpersonal

83

psychological phenomena. By bringing our curiosity to the models of yoga and psychology as a springboard for further studies, neuroscience is poised to explore the farther reaches of human nature.

Efficacy   Given the vast array of yogic and psychological methods, as well as the extensive time and resources required for effective research, it would be sensible to prioritize research on practices based on their efficacy—namely by identifying practices engaged in by a large number of people over a long period of time or practices across traditions with overlapping mechanisms and goals. Specifically, we are better served by prioritizing research on practices that have been traditionally or historically regarded as efficacious in achieving certain states of consciousness.

Blueprint for transformation   Modern medicine is currently building a robust understanding of the relationships between our biological and genetic makeup and states of illness and disease. What is yet to be developed is a map of the links between neurobiology and optimal health. We can use a collaborative investigation of the effects of yogic and psychological tools on the human nervous system, especially in the long term, to create such a blueprint for optimal health and transformational possibilities. This would offer a map of plausible possibilities for growth and well-being given the past and present states of an individual's nervous system. Furthermore, we can use discoveries in neuroscience as reference points to inform us how to navigate our personal and collective transformative journeys, converting otherwise technical information into practical knowledge. Creating a cartography of the interactions between the nervous system, yoga, and psychology will foster a transition to a greater living knowledge of ourselves.

Citizen science   Academic institutions are currently on the cutting edge of neuroscience research. The next phase currently gaining traction is the extension of research into the hands of ordinary citizens, making for a more democratized science. In learning to think scientifically, instructors and practitioners of yoga, mental-health practitioners and their clients, and all those interested in these fields can actively participate in the process of scientific discovery. Science is a process of asking a question about the unknown given a certain set of known factors. We are all capable of asking useful questions: What do we want to know? What is already known about it? What methods do we need to employ to find out what we want to know? And we can ask these at home, in the laboratory, on the yoga mat, in the workplace, or in a psychotherapy setting. Additionally, we're all capable of using or accessing qualitative measures such as question-naires in addition to more quantitative measures such as heart-rate variability and brain imaging. The sooner we transform a gap in knowledge into an open question, the more expeditiously the engine of scientific discovery becomes available for anyone to work in con-cert with others toward enhanced knowledge for us all.

Yoga, psychology, and neuroscience are synergistic disciplines, each contributing a crucial piece of the puzzle of optimal human func-tion. They inform each other such that what they generate as a whole becomes greater than the sum of their respective parts. Discovering the wonders of the brain can give stunning detail to yogic and psychologi-cal practices and has the potential to offer a more targeted guidance for practitioners, guides, teachers, and students alike. Neuroscience has the potential to illuminate our transformative paths, both individually and collectively, and we can turn the information derived from studies into practical knowledge. Through applying neuroscience to the inte-gration of yoga and psychology, we can transform the body, mind, and nervous system into one seamless evolutionary process that, for lovers of truth and self-knowledge, literally has no end.

6

HOW SOMATIC PSYCHOLOGY CHANGES THE GAME

*The separation of psychology from the premises of biology
is purely artificial, because the human psyche lives
in indissoluble union with the body.*[1]
CARL JUNG

"Y ou are *not* in your body," my therapist told me. I was mortified. If I was not in my body, where was I? And how could I get back into it? Was I the only one with this issue? My therapist had named the problem but didn't provide any answers. I felt ashamed, frustrated, and confused.

I was twenty-three at the time. I didn't truly take on the issue until a decade or so later. Although I had years of experience as a yoga practitioner, therapist, and client in psychotherapy, I still had not broken through some abiding patterns instigated by childhood trauma. I knew someone who was focusing his psychotherapy practice on using somatics with trauma, so I became his client. During our first session—when I was narrating the same old, familiar story of my life—my new therapist kept interrupting me with questions such as "And what are you feeling in your body as you describe that?" and "Where do you feel that emotion in your body?" I didn't know how to respond. I left that first session with an all-too-familiar sense of confusion.

However, I woke up the next morning feeling different—somehow more *alive*. With my therapist's compassionate guidance over the next few months, I finally began to feel the inside of my body and use the practices of somatics to make incredible discoveries. I got so much out of the experience that I promptly enrolled in Peter Levine's three-year training program in the Somatic Experiencing Method and began to explore other techniques of trauma and somatic healing. My work as a therapist—and my own embodied experience—has never been the same since.

Somatic psychology radically changes the game in that it introduces practical methods to understand psychological challenges and unwind stuck patterns and traumas through directly accessing knowledge and awareness in (and through) our bodies. When integrating and combining the advances in somatics with the exciting developments in neuroscience (and the growing intersection of neuroscience with psychology and yoga covered in chapter 5), we can further unwind our traumas, influence our karma, gain self-knowledge, and fulfill all the possibilities of what it means to be human.

THE EMERGENCE OF SOMATIC PSYCHOLOGY

Thomas Hanna first applied the term *somatics* to the field of psychology in the 1970s in a desire to merge the Western split between mind and body. He declared, "Soma does not mean 'body'; it means 'Me, the bodily being.'"[2] Hanna later defined somatics as, "The field which studies the soma: namely the body as perceived from within the first-person perception . . . the human being as experienced by himself [or herself] from the inside."[3] Recent approaches to somatic psychology and body-oriented psychotherapy include Somatic Experiencing, Sensorimotor Psychotherapy, Hakomi Method, Core Energetics, Bioenergetics, Body-Mind Centering, Somatic Trauma Therapy, Integrative Body Psychotherapy, Holotropic Breathwork, Core Energetics, and iRest. These approaches all offer methods to heal trauma and psychological wounds in body and mind, and some extend their scope to support individuals in self-actualization and thriving.

Somatic approaches work directly with present phenomena in the body and unwind psychological material via the means of direct experience. As Bill Bowen, the founder of Psycho-Physical Therapy, puts it:

> Body and mind work together. They are mutually influential and interactive. We call these integrative actions psycho-physical functioning: the combined interactions of body and mind. Because of this interconnected functioning, psychological issues affect the body and, conversely, the quality of physical interaction has an effect on psychological functioning. This concept is common knowledge in psychotherapeutic work but is often underutilized. To actively work from this concept means to continually look for and engage the interactive dynamics of mind and body in all stages of the therapeutic process.[4]

Through becoming more aware of the connection between bodily symptoms and emotions with the support of a knowledgeable and skillful therapist, clients become empowered to explore and release physical symptoms and psychological contractions in their own bodies. The body itself reveals insight, connections, and direction as to what adjustments to perspectives, choices, or habits the client needs to make. Studies support the effectiveness of somatic psychology in treating issues such as depression, which is increasingly being recognized as an ailment that requires addressing both mind and body for full recovery.[5] Body-therapy treatments, too, have been demonstrated to significantly improve symptoms of anxiety, interpersonal problems, and psychosomatic grievances, particularly when treatment occurs over a longer period of time.[6]

Most notably, somatic psychology is increasingly viewed in the field as one of the most effective treatments for various types of trauma, precisely because trauma impacts the nervous system so viscerally.[7] Numerous studies demonstrate that therapeutic techniques that include the body improve self-regulation, increase body awareness, reduce dissociation, foster self-care and pain-management skills, and allow for the body's innate wisdom to complete impulses that may have been halted during the time of the instigating traumatic event.[8]

SOMATIC PSYCHOTHERAPY: THERAPY FROM THE INSIDE OUT

By bringing somatics more directly into the therapeutic process, we discover the emotional language of our own body. In itself, the simple but profound process of learning to compassionately feel and experience our own bodies from the inside out is enough to change our lives. It is often said that the longest distance in the world is from the head to the heart. Yet even this connection is just the beginning of the journey into the body. Clients are regularly surprised at the power of learning to listen to their body in a new way and discover new methods for working with their trauma and unconscious patterns.

For example, Bill came to me for therapy complaining of severe contraction and discomfort in his body that traveled down his throat, through his heart, and into his belly. Despite spending thousands of dollars on medical treatments (mainstream and alternative), new exercise and diet regimes, and spiritual retreats, Bill's suffering persisted. By the time Bill hit his forties, he lived almost constantly with anxiety, insomnia, physical pain, and overall dissatisfaction with his life in spite of his numerous successes. As it turned out, Bill had suffered from perfectionism since childhood, seeking out validation for everything in his life, and endured unprocessed events—including the death of his sibling and a parent when he was a teen. I encouraged Bill to listen to the pains and contractions in his body. Bill learned to bring love to the impulses, images, stories, and everyday traumas contained within them, as well as to pay attention to the desires he had never allowed himself to listen to because they didn't align with the self-image of perfection he had always strived toward. As we listened to the profound exhaustion in his body, I gently suggested that he might need some deep rest in order to recover. "Wow," he said. "It truly never occurred to me that I might just need rest, and a lot of it."

Although it took a lot of courage to do so, Bill took an indefinite leave of absence from his job and went offline, traveled to the tropics, and allowed his body to rest while being nourished with massage, healthy food, and nature for several months. His symptoms improved, and Bill was able to discover a different line of work that brought him a sense of purpose and contribution to the world. Of course, not everyone can escape to the tropics in this way to heal their ailments. However, all of us can rely on the wisdom of the body itself to find answers to questions we may have spent years contemplating. Our bodies also offer a plethora of information about the deep psyche: our dreams, callings, desires, and hidden gifts. Paradoxically, it is often through the willingness to enter our wounds that we discover our most important gifts.

It is only in recent years that the field of somatics has begun to intersect with the field of yoga in any formal way. Both fields share a respect for the body as a vehicle for self-knowledge and healing. For those interested in blending the two, it's helpful to understand the various aspects of yoga (meditation, breathwork, visualization, and so on) in addition to having some grounding in psychological training. As this learning process can take several years, most programs that integrate somatics and yoga have not yet advanced beyond the initial stages of development.

Somatic psychology is not necessarily the best or only mode of therapy that I utilize and recommend. However, it can serve as a powerful revelatory tool when incorporated with other modalities of therapy—particularly yoga. Blending the two was life changing for me; I feel certain it will be for others, as well.

EMBODIMENT: THE AWAKENING OF BODY CONSCIOUSNESS

Most of us experience the locus of our consciousness somewhere in, around, or above our heads. Our attention bounces around and swirls in endless thoughts in a way that many of us feel powerless to control. This is what is meant by disembodiment. We might have moments of feeling our bodies during sex, intense exercise, yoga, enjoying food, falling in love, having our heart broken, or experiencing intense emotions, but these are typically fleeting moments. Most of the vast domain of the interior of our bodies remains unexplored and unknown. I once sat at the deathbed of someone dear to me; huge tumors grew throughout her body. As the cancer invaded everywhere, she spoke about how much she was now feeling deep inside her body. "I can't believe it," she marveled. "I have been living inside my body for so many years and never even felt it from inside until now." I vowed I would not wait a whole lifetime to get into my body and feel it from the inside out.

Embodiment refers to the awakening of consciousness in and throughout the body. Once we discover the key to unlocking the interior of our body—and the immense possibilities for feeling our lives more intimately and moving through our experience from a different place within ourselves—it is not a matter of being *in* or *out* of one's body, but rather an ongoing and progressive process of exploring the potential in the expanse of embodiment. I recall a conversation I had years ago with Reggie Ray, an American Buddhist teacher who has been exploring the relationship between the psyche and body for more than forty years. Reggie told me he had recently discovered an area of contracted consciousness in the back of the second toe on his left foot, and had been amazed at the consciousness and information that had opened up there. As I learned from my more experienced peer, the possibilities for exploring embodiment never end.

Few people were raised in environments in which their parents and caregivers modeled or taught them to listen to their body's innate wisdom. Instead, we grow up learning how to excessively think, eat, drink, override, overexert, and distract ourselves in a multitude of ways that keep us from knowing and feeling our bodies. In doing so, we also remain disconnected from others, from nature, and from the deeper body of the earth. Accordingly, we find disembodiment (consciously or unconsciously) as a safer option because we intuit that to open to the inner knowledge of the body means to open to the storehouses of feeling. Often this means engaging with trauma that may have been held within us for a lifetime—including the trauma suffered by others and the earth itself. Anodea Judith succinctly describes disembodiment in *Eastern Body, Western Mind*:

> Our culture, so proud of its mind-over-matter philosophy, cuts us off from our bodily experience and from the earth itself. In this severance, our sexuality is negated, our senses assaulted, our environment abused, and our power manipulated. Our ground is our form, and without it we lose our individuality. At the other end of the pole, misinformation and indoctrination invalidate our consciousness. The child who is told he did not see what he just saw or could not have felt what he was feeling learns to doubt his own awareness. Instincts and memories may become disconnected from the body. This can produce phobias and compulsive activity, where behavior does not necessarily match the intention of the conscious mind. Fortunately, information and experience are stored in both physical and mental states. When one side is cut off, the other side can often be accessed. Our bodies can recover memories our minds have forgotten . . . . To lose our connection with the body is to become spiritually homeless. Without an anchor we float aimlessly, battered by the winds and waves of life.[9]

As a long-term practitioner of yoga, it amazed me to discover that a person can be intimately connected to her or his physical body but have little or no awareness of the emotional body. People are continually surprised, understandably disillusioned, and sometimes badly hurt by so-called yoga masters who possess profound control over their physical bodies—some even to the point of transmitting powerful spiritual experiences and knowledge—yet who demonstrate fallibility with respect to issues of sexuality, emotional maturity, communication, power, finances, and control. Sometimes physical and spiritual mastery unconsciously serves as a clever defense mechanism against feeling the intensity of emotional wounding. People often come to yoga and other spiritual traditions with the conscious or unconscious hope that gaining control over their bodies or minds and accessing spiritual experiences will obviate the need to do the grittier and ongoing work of entering the world of emotions.

Therefore, when we begin to reinhabit our bodies, we may first discover pains and traumas that have been ignored for a lifetime. When people begin inner work for the first time, they may often feel worse, or at least feel *more*, before they begin to feel better as they encounter trauma embedded within their bodies. (Feeling worse can in some cases be avoided, with the help of a skilled therapist.) For some, the discovery of embodiment becomes more than a process of healing—it becomes a path itself, be it spiritual or psychological. For these people, embodiment means progressively opening the capacity to connect with one's own endless depths and with wonderment and appreciation for the ordinary magic in daily life. As trauma psychologist Peter Levine writes:

> Embodiment is about gaining, through the vehicle of
> awareness, the capacity to feel the ambient physical
> sensations of unfettered energy and aliveness as they
> pulse through our bodies. It is here that mind and
> body, thought and feeling, psyche and spirit, are
> held together, welded in an undifferentiated unity of
> experience. Through embodiment, we gain a unique
> way to touch into our darkest primitive instincts and
> to experience them as they play into the daylight dance
> of consciousness, and in so doing to know ourselves as
> though for the first time—in a way that imparts vitality,
> flow, color, hue, and creativity to our lives.[10]

When embodiment becomes a passion and way of life with endless possibilities, the world opens in surprising and meaningful ways. Whereas at one time the potential to experience our lives from our bodies may have been foreign and even frightening, living within our bodies becomes the safest and most connected way of inhabiting our experience.

DISCOVER YOUR INNER PHYSICIAN'S POWER OF SELF-HEALING

In Sanskrit, the name Jangalykayamane refers to the jungle physician or inner healer. As a deity in yogic philosophy, this principle represents our capacity to heal the various ailments of mind, body, and spirit. The inner physician within each of us is also responsible for wholeness and spiritual awareness. The yogis of old were not accompanied by medical professionals when they went into the forest to pursue spiritual realization. They had to learn to heal themselves by means of yogic practices—posture, breath, movement, purification, awareness, meditation, diet, and cleanses.

I was initially skeptical about the concept of an inner healer. It sounded overly New Agey and dubious to me. It was only my own three-year bout with a severe, undiagnosed immune disorder that enabled me to access my own inner healer. Through my own journey into almost complete remission, I discovered for myself that such a capacity exists within each and every one of us. We need only to find the guidance and support to access it, as well as the willingness to listen to it. This does not mean we can prevent or heal all illnesses, but we can access our inner healer to respond to whatever we are faced with. I often hear clients articulate a problem of theirs and then clearly present an appropriate healing response to that problem. Personally, when I am in a weakened or injured state of body or mind, if I listen closely enough my body knows precisely what it needs to get better, or at least what types of help to seek. One of my mentors, Robert Svoboda, often quotes his guru—the Aghori Vimalananda—as saying, "If you fail to live with reality, reality inevitably comes to live with you." When we don't listen to our bodies, our bodies scream louder and louder—whether through fatigue, breakdown, or physical and psychological illness.

The principle of the inner physician effectively bridges both fields of somatics and yoga. When drawing upon the insights and practices of both traditions and the continual advances in trauma research and neuroscience, we become empowered to effectively heal ourselves and to know what kinds of external support we need.

Somatic psychology helps us to access psychological material from the inside out. And those who develop a mature yoga practice can eventually use the various aspects of yoga to gain access to their inner experience and make subtle but profound adjustments to their body, thoughts, breath, and nervous system. In this way, the practitioner discovers yoga from within, enabling them to follow the wisdom of their inner healer, relying less on the directives of external sources.

Through much trial and error, I have learned to help clients access their own inner physician. Through their own intuition and inner wisdom, my clients know more about their optimal healing journey than I do. As I've mentioned before, realizations that come from clients themselves are far more potent and lasting than those presented by an external source—in this case, me, the therapist. When we discover our own capacity to listen to our bodies in this way, we emerge with an enduring sense of empowerment. We come to trust our inner physician and revel in our capacity to heal ourselves.

THE TANTRIC PERSPECTIVE: A GOLDEN LINK

"One reaches heaven by the very things which may lead to hell," says an ancient tantric text called the Kularnava Tantra. The tantric perspective connects the fields of somatics and yoga like a golden link. Unfortunately, what we in the West think of when we hear the word *tantra* is often limited to esoteric, mystical sex. True, tantra includes sexuality, but the tantric path views all of life as fertile grounds for integrated spiritual transformation. Translated as "continuity," "fabric," "to weave," "technique," "method," and "nonrejection," tantra teaches us to knit the totality of our experience—good and bad, dark and light, spiritual and unspiritual—into one continuous fabric of awakened awareness.

Tantra is most overtly found in Hinduism and Buddhism, but tantric principles can also be found in Jewish Kabbalah, mystical Christianity, Sufism, some martial arts, and certain approaches to somatics and psychology. These approaches share a recognition that spiritual transformation lies within the everyday stuff of life. Rather than attempting to transcend and rise above our human experience, tantra encourages us to move in and through life. Although we may naturally prefer pleasant, blissful, and expansive experiences—and those on a yogic path are often more prone to prioritizing these over others—the tantric perspective encourages us to look at all of life as a transformational theater.

I recall a conversation I had with Robert Beer, a dear friend who is an amazing artist and foremost scholar of Tibetan and Nepali *thangka* paintings. Thangkas frequently depict Hindu and Buddhist deities and are often used in tantric visualization practices. I had been collecting paintings for some time, and due to my lifelong interest in examining the shadow sides of the psyche, I was particularly interested in the so-called wrathful deities that are fiercely depicted with multiple arms, heads, weapons, and so forth. I asked Robert whether he thought my inclination toward these darker expressions of divinity was problematic. He paused before answering. With a quizzical look, Robert replied, "Dark? Light? These are *all* expressions of the divine. There is nothing that is not divinity."

The tantric perspective excludes nothing from the domain of transformation. It values immanence—in this world—as well as transcendence. Tantra even suggests that the exploration of one enhances the discovery of the other. It advocates that enlightenment is not found just by moving toward the light, or by even mindfully observing the dark, but by moving toward and through obscurations as a way of opening to awareness and light. Those of us familiar with asana practice do this when we bring our breath, attention, and curious awareness to the contracted sensations, emotions, and energies in our bodies. By allowing them to simply be there, our acceptance releases tensions and may even open us up to welcome experiences of pleasure, energy, and spaciousness.

Mother Teresa of Calcutta said, "If I ever become a saint—I will surely be one of 'darkness.' I will continually be absent from heaven—to light the light of those in darkness on earth."[11] The tantric path of transformation is not for everybody; turning toward the more obscured, shadow sides of our experience can prove scary and challenging. However, with the support of somatics, neuroscience, mindfulness, and trauma therapies, tantra can serve as a seamless link between yoga and Western psychology. Following are some key ways it does so and why.

Tantra Emphasizes the Body in Transformation

When we embrace a tantric perspective in conjunction with the gifts of somatic psychology, the body becomes the true laboratory in which transformation is experienced and expressed. Embodiment and the discovery of the true sacredness of one's own body become essential to our spiritual development. Although contemporary yogic approaches may work with the body, too many still aim to paradoxically use the body to transcend human experience. Although universal in their essence, many yogic traditions present a transcendent perspective that inherently negates a feminine, embodied approach that includes sexuality, birth, death, emotions, and other organic processes that constitute the embodied human experience.

From a tantric perspective, sensuality, sexuality, and the senses are not distractions from transformation. Rather, they can serve as the very means of exploring, experiencing, and expressing transformation. In my experience with clients, spiritual teachers, and practitioners around the world, I've seen far too much renunciation and repression of the body—particularly sexuality—in service of transformation. People have various reasons for committing this error. Some think it's the "yogic way," some are following (or misinterpreting) the instructions of their teachers, and some are acting out of inherited notions of sin and impurity. Regardless, this type of negation—especially when it comes to sexuality—has ultimately caused more harm than good, in addition to being fraught with the pitfalls of spiritual bypassing discussed in chapter 2. As Greek author Nikos Kazantzakis writes:

> Within me even the most metaphysical problem takes on a
> warm, physical body which smells of sea, soil, and human sweat.
> The Word, in order to touch me, must become warm flesh.
> Only then do I understand—when I can smell, see, touch.[12]

By turning toward the body in this way—moving through its subsequent layers of psychological conditioning with an aim to eventually embrace its sacredness—the tantric approach, in conjunction with the brilliance of somatic practice, offers a life-affirming, down-to-earth, and practical approach to transformation.

Tantra Includes the Emotional Body as Grounds for Transformation

Tantra recognizes that emotion is a quintessential aspect of human experience. Furthermore, it asserts that powerful emotions themselves contain storehouses of healing life force that we can harness when we tune into these experiences with skillful awareness.

Over the years, clients have come to me feeling frustrated and disheartened that their extensive yogic and meditation practices—sometimes decades long—have not brought them consistent peace and spaciousness. They avidly began their pursuit of spirituality thinking that if they worked hard enough or practiced long enough, their challenging emotions would somehow disappear into the light of awareness. This is neither a realistic nor a desirable outcome. The spiritual teachers and masters I have met who claim to have transcended emotional experience have come across as flat and one-dimensional to me. Even among those who appear to have succeeded in transcending their emotions, the transformation is certainly lopsided; most likely what they consider spiritual metamorphosis is merely a form of unrecognized repression. These people may have awoken one aspect of their full humanity, but so much else—including the murky waters of human emotionality—remains fragmented and unaddressed. As Chögyam Trungpa Rinpoche notes:

> The chaos that takes place in your neurosis is the
> only home ground that you can build the mandala of
> awakening on. If we are looking for something else, then
> we want to reject that ground and find a better, higher
> place. If we are looking for an ideal spot, we never find it.

99

> Large areas of our life have been devoted to trying to avoid
> discovering our own experience. Now we have a chance
> to explore that large area which exists in our being, which
> we have been trying to avoid. That seems to be the first
> message, which may be very grim, but also very exciting.[13]

When we combine the insights of trauma research and neuroscience with the methods of somatics, and then place this merger in the context of tantra, we can work skillfully with our emotions and mine them for their transformational gifts. This is also the juncture where the refined tools of psychology can help us uncover, examine, and work with the challenges and promises of our emotions.

Tantra Teaches How to Transform Psychological Challenges into Gifts

Tantric practice teaches us to turn poison into medicine. According to this perspective, we do not need to throw away any aspect of ourselves, including those parts we most dislike and fear. If we use these facets, we gain energy from them and grow; if we misuse them, they deplete us and increase our confusion.

Even if they appear to be simple, every human being is unique, possessing incredible psychological complexity and intensity. Some yogic teachings assert that our psychological makeup is, in essence, unreal. Other potent meditation techniques teach us how to observe certain aspects of our psychological experience and cultivate an attitude of detachment when they arise so that these facets cease to dominate our experience. I think these techniques only work for some people some of the time. Rarely do they stand the test of intimate relationship and sexuality. As the adage goes, "If you want to know how enlightened someone is, ask their spouse/partner."

In contrast, both tantra and somatics differ in that they teach that the cure for a wound comes from turning toward it. When we pay attention to that which we ordinarily hide from, we establish a relationship with it and thereby engage its energetic makeup with conscious awareness, release blocked energy, and allow previously unknown aspects of our experience to inform and heal us. Tantra teaches us to investigate the gold mine of confused experience and extract the pure energy of the life force contained therein. From this perspective, our neurosis is not a limitation. Instead, we limit ourselves when we contract and turn away from experiences that scare us with their sensitivity and potency—wounds so tender that we repress them from conscious awareness and fears so convincing that we would rather live restricted lives than open ourselves to them.

Working in a tantric way requires using our awareness and attention differently. We don't necessarily stop having strong emotions or even stop being neurotic (at least not right away), but our attention and intention refocus these in the service of transformation. Although part of us continues to enact the same conditioned behaviors of daily life—eating breakfast, freaking out, working, being confused, doing our best to love while falling short of the mark—our basic orientation slowly turns toward transformation. Over time, particularly when supported with depth psychology and somatics, we co-opt our so-called weaknesses into the service of a greater reality. Doing so, we escape the stranglehold of our neurosis and channel that energy into our own creativity and growth.

I once invited Robina Courtin, an Australian-born teacher of Tibetan Buddhism, to lecture on tantra to a group of graduate students. Robina told them she had been an "angry, Marxist, radical, lesbian biker-chick" before meeting her spiritual teacher. Decades later, she still experienced anger, but she was able to use it toward social justice causes—among them, teaching Buddhism to convicts in maximum-security prisons. Robina's lifelong sense of not belonging anywhere turned into a life of teaching around the world, and her anxiety and restlessness resulted in the creation of a number of spiritual centers and large-scale service projects. She had learned to transform her personal challenges into assets, not only for herself but also for others, thereby benefitting thousands of people who are touched by her presence.

Robina's example is more extreme than most of our lives, but it does demonstrate the primary point—we can actually engage the more difficult aspects of our experience for the greater good, and all the more so when we integrate tantra, psychology, somatics, yoga, and other embodiment practices.

Contentment, Pleasure, and Joy Come Back Online

In the years I spent living in an ashram in my twenties, I always found it challenging that austerities and renunciation were overemphasized, whereas simple pleasures, joy, and relaxation were considered indulgent. I received an underlying message that financial abundance, physical pleasure, play, and personal contentment were questionable and to be frowned upon. Far too many yogic paths consider life as something requiring transcendence. In contrast, when we combine the skillful means of tantric yoga with psychology's emphasis on understanding and healing, we can bring contentment, pleasure, and joy back into our lives. By embracing life-affirming paths to transformation that include all aspects of our experience, we claim all of life as the grounds of our spiritual life and the only place where abiding contentment and happiness can be found.

When I explore inner work with myself or my clients, I want results on all levels—I want to see more success relationally, vocationally, and spiritually. Additionally, I want to unleash more happiness and pleasure in our lives. When we discover joy—even ecstasy—and learn to experience it alongside the varieties of our inevitable suffering, we can actually become true agents of healing and happiness for ourselves and others.

Our Inner Work Results in Serving Something Greater

Although not explicitly described in many ancient texts, the tantric perspective expressed in the context of the modern world inevitably leads to the desire and increased capacity to make a difference in the world, whether expressed through parenting, community-oriented endeavors, social-justice work, or environmental advocacy. The challenges we face as a species and as a collective that includes the planet itself are undeniable at this point. We need a tantric perspective, therefore, that not only includes all aspects of our experience, but those of the earth and our fellow creatures as well.

Practicing tantra heightens our connection to other manifestations of life; therefore, our need to contribute naturally grows. It has been amply documented anecdotally and scientifically that service to others brings increased happiness to oneself. People often want to make a contribution, but they either feel they don't have anything to offer or they don't know how to share their gifts. When we integrate tantra and psychology, we call forth our inner resources and recognize our unique gifts, enabling us to activate our desire and capacity to help others.

SOMATICS + TANTRA = EXPANDED TOOLS FOR EMBODIMENT

Although the reaches of tantra extend far beyond those ordinarily aspired to by somatic psychology, both fields respect the body and consider the individual's present experience as the primary ground for transformation. Each excels in a different arena. Somatics—particularly when combined with advances in neuroscience and trauma therapies—offers skills and tools to address the traumas that so commonly afflict the Western psyche. On the other hand, tantra provides an extensive array of embodied practice including meditation, visualization, mantra, sexual practices, pranayama, partner work, deity practices, and much more. The perspective gained through tantra empowers the practitioner to engage an endless exploration into the inner and outer realms of life that is directed from the wisdom of the body.

Practicing asana while embracing these two perspectives allows transformation to "pop" within the body as we peel away layers of obscuration and meet them with the diamond-like, integrated awareness of tantra and somatics. Through this level of spiritual practice, we experience a profound connectedness to something greater. This, in turn, enables us to penetrate the delicate, folded layers of the psyche that contain our wounding and even our ancient karmic conditioning. When we unlock the contracted energies held within our wounds, trauma, shame, and self-hatred, it frees up tremendous life force that fuels our spiritual practice. In this way, these practices together form a transformational path that is simultaneously mystical, embodied, and pragmatic. The possibilities for endless embodiment are literally at our fingertips.

In summary, from a tantric perspective, yogic transformation doesn't mean leaving behind this world, our bodies, our relationships, or anything else. We bring everything to the table, which is why psychology becomes so relevant. Tantra doesn't ask us to leave ourselves at the door and pretend we are someone else. Quite the contrary. When we engage tantric practice optimally—especially when we utilize somatics—we can turn our most painful wounds into our brightest gifts.

OVERCOMING TRAUMA
WITH SOMATICS
AND YOGA

We can get past the slipperiness of words by engaging the self-observing, body-based self system, which speaks through sensations, tone of voice, and body tensions. Being able to perceive visceral sensations is the very foundation of emotional awareness.[1]
BESSEL VAN DER KOLK

How can I feel so bad if nothing terrible ever happened to me?" It's a question that new clients frequently bring to therapy. I also hear it uttered in the hearts of so many who pursue yoga and spiritual practice in the attempt to alleviate sufferings that have no name or apparent source. Countless people push down their emotions and negate the validity of their inner challenges for much of their lives because they do not think the feelings are justified, especially when others have suffered so much worse. Or maybe as children they were told they were given everything they needed, even though what they most needed was a certain kind of care, attention, or mirroring they never received. Some people come to therapy believing that they must uncover a specific memory or causal reason to legitimize their pain and body memories, even though such may have occurred before they were able to form concepts and words to understand them.

Every human being alive experiences a full spectrum of feeling. Every human life possesses a certain intensity. When visiting rural Guatemalan churches, I witnessed destitute people praying out loud at simple altars. I was moved by their lack of shame and their full and unrepressed expression of what they had been through, the sorrows they carried, and their heartfelt petitions for health, happiness, and abundance for themselves and their loved ones. Because I know Spanish, I listened to their profound pleas for world peace and the end of political suffering in Guatemala, as well as their laments for those lost to war and sickness, their pinings for their deceased, and their longings for love so universal among all peoples.

Just as colors exist on a spectrum in relationship to each other and combine to make all hues seen and unseen, we cannot experience the full dimensionality of our embodied experience without anger, sorrow, joy, fear, contentment, and the endless subtleties and complexities of emotions that lie somewhere on the continuum of experience. These feelings do not arise because something is wrong with us but rather because we are alive. Accordingly, one of our tasks as living beings is learning how to relate to our emotions, whether we have experienced severe traumas in childhood or simply the everyday traumas that are inescapable in today's world.

REDEFINING TRAUMA

For good reason, the subject of trauma has received significant attention in recent years, and a number of new therapies have been created to address it. Trauma theory gives a language and context for the suffering that so many people experience. Although we can look at trauma through various viewpoints, for the purposes of this chapter we'll focus on everyday trauma, childhood and developmental trauma, the diagnostic categories of the clinically recognized post-traumatic stress disorder (PTSD), and the increasingly acknowledged complex post-traumatic stress disorder (or complex trauma). However, I also want to note that the distinctions between types of trauma often overlap, that they occur on a spectrum of intensity, and that people experience traumas in ways genuinely unique to them. Before we explore further, I think it's helpful to keep in mind that trauma catalysts include a wide array of events: physical, emotional, or sexual abuse in childhood or adulthood; emotionally abusive relationships; harassment, bullying, and domestic violence; racial abuse and discrimination; employment discrimination; abandonment, rejection, and codependence; judicial corruption and misconduct; indoctrination; being the child of an alcoholic parent; the threat of violence or witnessing violence; life-threatening medical conditions and medication-induced trauma; catastrophic natural disasters such as earthquakes, tornadoes, and volcanic eruptions; transportation accidents; fire; mass interpersonal violence such as war and terrorist attacks; sex trafficking; and being taken as a hostage or kidnapped. Additionally, long-term exposure to extreme poverty, psychological and verbal abuse, and psychological manipulation are examples of traumas that are not physical but still generate psychological trauma.

Leading researchers, doctors, and psychologists alike recognize that trauma and its impact are most effectively defined by a person's response rather than the intrinsic nature of the event itself. This critical insight explains how two children of the same family can be exposed to similar violence or poor parenting and one child ends up much more wounded, or the two children are impacted in very different ways. Likewise, one victim of a major car accident may experience no symptoms of PTSD whereas another person in the same accident—or in a less serious accident—may suffer from flashbacks, shakiness, hypervigilance, and other symptoms that endure for years. Our individual psyches and bodies have distinct constitutions, and they are informed by all of our experiences in this life—and perhaps those of preceding generations.

In his book *The Body Bears the Burden: Trauma, Dissociation, and Disease*, leading trauma researcher Robert Scaer writes:

> Stress may be defined in one sense as any negative stimulus that produces persistent activation of the sympathetic nervous system and related HPA [hypothalamic–pituitary–adrenal axis] pathways. Trauma may be viewed in this light as an extreme form of stress, one that has assumed life-threatening proportions.[2]

In other words, any stressors that produce classic trauma symptoms such as flashbacks, re-experiencing, avoidance, or somatic arousal can realistically be described as a traumatic event, regardless of exactly what happened or even whether or not it is remembered. What may be mildly upsetting for one individual is outright devastating for another, and that is significantly determined by many factors including the individual's prior life experience, any other previous traumatic event(s) that remind them of the current event, and the meaning they make of the inciting stressor.

People remember trauma in varying ways, directly and indirectly. As a psychotherapist, I've come to appreciate the subtleties of these differences:

- **Preverbal memories** occur before we understand language (for example, mistreatment during infancy or a depressed parent).

- **Precognitive memories** form when we lack the concepts or framework to understand events (for example, a child whose parents divorce when they are young or who is raised in a climate of unspoken marital tension).

- **Emotional memories** can be stored without images or constructs (for example, someone who experiences fears at night without remembering anything specifically traumatic happening at night, or a child who was raised in a climate of chronic, functional alcoholism or addiction).

- **Somatic memories** arise as strong sensations in the body (for example, feeling hypervigilant without a specific reason or experiencing intense physical alarm when hearing someone scream).

These types of traumatic memory tend to overlap and blur within the psyche and express themselves in unexpected and often nonlinear ways. Particularly when we experience trauma as children, it might not register until we experience affiliated circumstances as adults, and even then the connection between our experience and the event may be hidden. In this case, we might become inexplicably upset in strange situations or feel unable to control our reactions even when they are unhealthy and self-sabotaging.

When people can't directly remember traumatic events, they often deny themselves the right to their accompanying feelings and, therefore, the possibility of resolving the trauma. Seeking explanations, clinicians and clients alike sometimes make the mistake of trying to dig into or pummel the psyche for traumatic memories, often leading to futile and even misleading outcomes. False memories are a controversial topic in psychology, and they're addressed by Peter A. Levine, PhD, in his book *Trauma and Memory*. After a couple of decades in the field, here's what I've come to believe: Our feelings are valid and worthy of exploration simply because we feel them. Furthermore, we can make tremendous strides in our healing by learning to respect, turn toward, and intelligently process the images, emotions, and sensations within our bodies without having to know—literally or linearly—everything that has happened to us.

THE PERVASIVENESS OF EVERYDAY TRAUMA IN CONTEMPORARY CULTURE

The term *everyday trauma* refers to the inevitable pain and trauma that are experienced simply as a part of life—what Buddhism calls *dukkha*, or suffering. I regularly see everyday trauma in my practice: clients suffer from existential terror, the fear of death, loneliness, lack of purpose or fulfillment, and the remnants of painful childhood patterning even in the absence of severe trauma. People also experience the impact of collective trauma (for example, the current state of world politics or dread for the environment) even when they themselves are not immediately affected.

People also experience trauma with respect to things that have *not* happened: the longing for love and intimate partnership and the accompanying fear that such may never come (or return), the intense desire to have a child without the circumstances to support it (or missing the chance to be a parent), or regrets about opportunities missed and roads not taken earlier in life. Sometimes it's the things that didn't happen—rather than things that did—that bring such suffering that they can rightfully be classified as traumatic events. A woman with a terminal illness who will die before she is ready, a man with a life-threatening condition who has never known true friendship or love, a parent estranged from a child (or vice versa), someone who feels like their life is hurtling by without meaning. The suffering of everyday life takes endless forms.

The speed and complexity of today's world also play a crucial role. A surprising number of people report everyday trauma as a result of the repeated rejection and awkwardness inherent in online dating or from the plummeting self-esteem that results from comparing their lives to others' on social media. People whose organic rhythms are more attuned to the slower movements found in nature can become overstimulated and jarred in an accelerated world that requires multitasking. Those who are sensitive may also feel overwhelmed when around people who are psychologically immature, dense, or armored. In these ways and countless others, modern society intersects with our psycho-biological constitution and personal pasts to heighten our experience of everyday trauma. As Scaer notes, "As a result, even minor, nonviolent societal trauma should not be dismissed as a source of significant trauma in selected populations, especially if it occurs in a climate of relative helplessness and is out of one's control."[3]

Very few people are unaffected by everyday trauma. Trauma of all kinds occurs on a spectrum, but we experience symptoms in varying intensity at different points in our lives. Everyday trauma even arises in parents when their children go through particular stages of development, and even more so when the parent suffered a traumatic event as child at that particular age. Accordingly, although distinctions in types and degrees of trauma are useful to help indicate the most effective treatment, traumatic symptoms require attention and validation even in people who have no rational, linear explanation for their suffering.

CHILDHOOD AND DEVELOPMENTAL TRAUMA

The most well-documented area of trauma regards events that happened in childhood. Again, trauma is informed both by what happened to us (for example, physical abuse) and what didn't (lack of gestures of affection). Researchers assert that childhood trauma is rampant in the West. Pioneering trauma researcher Bessel van der Kolk notes:

> Childhood trauma, including abuse and neglect, is probably our nation's single most important public-health challenge, a challenge that has the potential to be largely resolved by appropriate prevention and intervention.
> Each year over three million children are reported to the authorities for abuse and/or neglect in the United States, of which about one million are substantiated. Many thousands more undergo traumatic medical and surgical procedures or are victims of accidents and of community violence. However, most trauma begins at home: the vast majority of people (about 80 percent) responsible for child maltreatment are the children's own parents.[4]

As it is described here, trauma has implications on the ability to form healthy attachments (in childhood and adulthood), emotional and behavioral regulation, dissociation, self-esteem, disease and health, and psychological well-being. Additionally, people who suffer childhood and developmental trauma are predisposed to addiction, anxiety, depression, insomnia, attention deficit hyperactivity disorder (ADHD), oppositional defiant disorder (ODD), and eating disorders. As van der Kolk notes above, this type of trauma is our country's greatest challenge to public health.

Hidden traumas from childhood can prove the most difficult to process. As noted above, these traumas often don't have names, concepts, or specific memories attached to them, and so far too many go undetected and untreated. Children internalize events they are incapable of understanding—undiagnosed psychopathology in parents, marital tensions, financial anxiety, grief, loneliness, the countless challenges facing immigrants, generational trauma (for example, that passed down from survivors of genocide), and so on.

Regarding the trauma of things that *did not happen*, I recall as a young child struggling with questions about death, love, religious hypocrisy, and the hurt I felt from some of my parents' behaviors. When I was in first grade I learned that the sun would one day burn out and that our entire planet would be subsequently obliterated, including every living thing on it. This discovery shook me to the core, and I suffered several years of anxiety and insomnia just thinking about our inevitable destruction. As a result, I was continually told, "You think too much," when all I really needed was some mirroring, understanding, and emotional empathy. Human development expert Joseph Chilton Pearce speaks to this when he refers to the absence of something that "was supposed to happen, but didn't." As children, what's supposed to happen is that our intense feelings, fears, exuberance, and brightness are met with care and love. Far too often, this doesn't happen, mostly because parents never received what was supposed to happen themselves, and they lack the awareness to process their own emotional struggles.

When traumas are not remembered at the level of ordinary memory or associated with a particular event, they are nearly impossible to resolve through conventional talk therapy alone. As we'll see later in this chapter, trauma that is felt and encoded in the body is best addressed through yoga and other somatic therapies in combination with psychotherapeutic modalities.

TRAUMA SYMPTOMS

Symptoms of trauma in children and adults include sleep disturbance, shock, achy muscles, stomachaches, lack of appetite, clinging to parents, social withdrawal, increased sensitivity, panic attacks, fatigue, lack of motivation, distraction, fidgeting, impulsivity, physical weakness, rapid heartbeat, fearfulness, emotionality (for example, cries easily), anger, aggressiveness, and flashbacks. These symptoms fall on a spectrum of severity as well as range in the degree to which they are recognized and considered legitimate.

PTSD refers to a set of stressors and resulting symptoms recognized by the DSM, and in order to be diagnosed with PTSD a person must be re-experiencing symptoms, displaying avoidance and numbing, and suffering arousal symptoms, with these all lasting at least one month. Re-experienced symptoms include persistent and uninvited memories of the event, nightmares, and emotional and somatic flashbacks. These may occur in unexpected moments and cause distress equivalent to (or reminiscent of) how the person felt during the event itself. Avoidance and numbing symptoms include detachment from others, repression, and the efforts people make to avoid remembering the event: staying away from particular places, sounds, or smells that remind them of the event. Finally, arousal symptoms include hypervigilance, difficulty concentrating, irritability, increased temper or anger, difficulty falling or staying asleep, and being easily startled. Still other common symptoms of PTSD (though not requisite for a diagnosis) include guilt, shame, self-blame, physical pain, suicidal ideation, depression, anxiety, feelings of distrust, helplessness, and a sense of betrayal.

Often when we become familiar with the signs of trauma, we discover that most of us know people—if not ourselves—who experience these symptoms. Sometimes our traumatic responses aren't triggered until decades after the instigating event. When we faced traumatic events as children, most of us did not have people around us to empathically support us through the pain and help us process our emotional and somatic reactions. If our parents and caregivers were repeatedly exposed to trauma in their own childhoods, critical parts of them remain frozen in time at certain levels of their development. Accordingly, they act out as children of that age when emotionally triggered—even well into adulthood and old age.

However, not everyone who experiences trauma develops PTSD or complex trauma. Body psychotherapist Babette Rothschild, MSW, writes:

> There is a mistaken assumption that anyone experiencing
> a traumatic event will develop PTSD. This is far from
> true. Results of studies vary but in general confirm that
> only a fraction of those facing such incidents—around 20

percent—will develop PTSD. What distinguishes those who do not is still a controversial topic, but there are many clues. Nonclinical factors that mediate traumatic stress appear to include preparation for expected stress (when possible), successful fight-or-flight response, developmental history, belief system, prior experience, internal resources, and support (from family, community, and social networks).[5]

When we experience somatic memories, flashbacks, and other ongoing symptoms of past trauma, our nervous system activates the fight/flight/freeze reaction, which is accompanied by various responses such as dissociating, collapsing, dodging, and bracing. The fight-or-flight response means that the sympathetic nervous system is experiencing hyperarousal, which includes symptoms such as accelerated heart rate, increased blood pressure, choppy breathing, jumpiness, cold sweat, sudden heat, darting eyes, and a general feeling of agitation and vigilance in relationship to one's environment. Longer-term consequences of hyperarousal can include ongoing anxiety and relational challenges, as well as chronic autoimmune disorders, insomnia, and gut issues, among other physiological responses due to the chronic activation of the sympathetic nervous system. Unfortunately, these consequences result in another insidious form of suffering. As Peter Levine writes:

> Because these sensations feel so dreadful [i.e., the physiological responses to trauma, including knots in the gut, rumbling gastrointestinal tract, tightness/suffocation in the lungs] they themselves become the source of threat. So rather than coming from outside, the threat now emanates from deep within one's bowels, lungs, heart, and other organs and can cause the exact same effect upon the viscera that the original threat once evoked . . . In addition, because traumatized individuals are experiencing (intense) threat signals, they project this inner turmoil outward and thus perceive the world as being responsible for their inner distress—and so remove themselves from both the real source of the problem and its potential

solution. This dynamic also wreaks havoc not only on the body but also on relationships.[6]

On the other hand, the autonomic nervous system can also respond with hypoarousal—parasympathetic responses that decrease physiological arousal. When we can't access our typical fight-or-flight responses during trauma, we may shut down, dissociate (check out or space out), or even freeze—also known as tonic immobility. The silent scream that occurs during intense fear or in nightmares (in which people try to scream but can't make any sound) is this type of parasympathetic response. Hypoarousal also takes the form of compromised digestion and immunity, depression, emotional shutting down, confusion, numbing, hypersomnia (excessive sleeping), social avoidance, fatigue and low energy, and feeling stuck in angry or sad emotions.

People sometimes experience overlapping and alternating sympathetic and parasympathetic responses due to ongoing dysregulation, switching between feeling shut down and disconnected from themselves and others, and then becoming hypersensitive and easily triggered. Yoga and somatic therapies are immensely helpful in teaching us to regulate sympathetic and parasympathetic arousal in our own bodies—particularly when we learn which practices are most effective—in addition to the most beneficial ways in which to engage them.

COMPLEX TRAUMA

Complex post-traumatic stress disorder (C-PTSD), also called complex trauma, is not yet recognized as a subcategory of trauma by the DSM. It refers to a series of symptoms that arise as the result of prolonged stress of a social nature, especially in the context of interpersonal dependence. Complex trauma arises when people suffer psychological manipulation, chronic maltreatment by primary caregivers, or sexual abuse and incest; or survive war, detention in a concentration camp, or belonging to a religious cult. It also arises when a person has had multiple kinds of trauma, resulting in layers of interwoven causes and symptoms that are challenging to tease apart. In my work, I have encountered a number of spiritual leaders, yoga teachers, and practitioners who suffer from complex trauma. In some cases, an early (usually unconscious) history of unresolved complex trauma draws them to their spiritual path.

Leading researchers on the forefront of trauma treatment—Peter Levine and Bessel van der Kolk, among others—distinguish the subtleties involved in diagnosing and caring for complex trauma. As van der Kolk writes:

> While PTSD has become the central organizing diagnosis for traumatized patients, it does not take into account the complexity of adaptation to trauma, nor does a patient's PTSD score inform clinicians about such relevant issues as functional impairment, developmental aspects of the trauma, what resources the patient has available to deal with their PTSD symptoms, and how different traumatizing life events have coalesced to give rise to the current clinical picture.[7]

The value of resources—financial, personal, and intellectual—when coping with trauma is apparent to those of us who work in the field. Clients can more readily heal themselves when they can articulate their trauma, know which treatments to explore, possess the financial resources required, and have the support of family and friends. Unfortunately, those who suffer from complex trauma are often marginalized in some way, and far too many lack access to these resources. For this reason, yoga and other open-source practices (once initially learned) are incredibly valuable for underserved populations.

SOMATIC HEALING FOR REGULATING THE NERVOUS SYSTEM

We don't need to remain victims of our trauma. Working through it can prove difficult and take years, but we now have multiple options to help us unravel and heal our particular sufferings. Specifically, research and anecdotal evidence demonstrate that somatically oriented therapies and yoga provide some of the most effective treatments for healing trauma, particularly by enabling a practitioner to regulate their own nervous system. I'll expound on some techniques to modulate nervous arousal and process trauma in the next chapter. The good news is that with proper guidance, we can use our own bodies to unwind trauma far more successfully than just employing traditional methods. As van der Kolk writes:

> The challenge of recovery [from trauma] is to reestablish
> ownership of your body and your mind—of your self.
> This means feeling free to know what you know and
> to feel what you feel without becoming overwhelmed,
> enraged, ashamed, or collapsed.[8]

Trauma is held within the body, and that's where it is ultimately resolved. The crucial initial steps of healing traumatic events often involve talking it through—particularly if the trauma arises from events that have left shame or secrecy in their wake, as is often the case in childhood abuse and sex-related traumas, as well as any type of trauma that leaves us believing we have done something bad or wrong. Speaking out the secrecy, understanding shame and its pervasive impact, and receiving empathic mirroring, care, and understanding from a qualified professional often brings relief, comfort, and even significant healing. When trauma is trapped by shame and secrecy, having our experience and symptoms understood and normalized often allows us to regain a sense of returning to the human race and helps us cease pathologizing ourselves.

However, trauma isn't just a memory of something that happened in the past. Trauma is a visceral imprint that remains in the body in the present moment. Our physiology is changed by trauma—it alters our feelings about ourselves and the way we experience the flow of sensation. For example, one of my clients was the victim of a date rape. It shattered her self-esteem, destroyed her sense that it is safe to follow her passions, and left her with chronic pains in her gut and chest. We began by addressing her secrecy, shame, and identity crisis, but it wasn't until we compassionately engaged the sensations, emotions, and memories trapped in her body that she rediscovered a sense of safety, along with the capacity to self-soothe and feel pleasure. Insight into and understanding of past experiences by themselves don't change the intensity of the ongoing, visceral persistence of trauma symptoms. People often find themselves at the door of a somatic therapist because even after years of talk therapy, the impact of trauma—including everyday trauma—continues to impede their full capacity for healing, transformation, and joy.

Even after engaging traditional therapies in a heartfelt way, people can still unconsciously play out their traumas in relationships despite their sincere efforts to do otherwise—for example, when people who were abused by parents or caregivers continue to find themselves in abusive intimate relationships well into adulthood. One way that a somatic approach to trauma would understand this unconscious replication is as the nervous system's patterning itself to a certain level of intensity. The person becomes neurologically rigged to expect a certain type and level of intensity, no matter how uncomfortable or unfulfilling. We can view the relational repetition as an impersonal function of the nervous system to reenact what it knows. Because trauma remains so little understood and recognized in its pervasiveness, many people who lack the resources (awareness, finances, or courage) to address their trauma will continue to enact the painful but familiar known experience over and over again, rather than begin the long journey of healing that trauma.

On the other hand, we can also view the tendency to repeat behaviors and relationships that reflect trauma as a recurring opportunity to heal. Each time we find ourselves in a painful but familiar situation, we have the chance to see—and more importantly feel—that which we may not have had the courage to face before. We also have the possibility to end the repetition of trauma, regulate our nervous system, and move toward healing, health, and thriving. Effective therapy therefore includes not only awareness and insight, but also the capacity to regulate emotion and transform previous life-negating patterns by consciously enacting new behaviors in the place of old ones. Sincere clients can actually integrate somatic awareness, psychotherapy, and yoga (especially its meditative focus and breathwork) to move through trauma in ways not previously imagined.

THE IMPORTANCE OF PACING

In my early years as a therapist, I worked with clients in underserved populations who were in severe crisis. As a new and inspired student of somatics and trauma, I was often overeager to help them get into their bodies, and my efforts regularly backfired. When we feel too much too soon without first feeling a sense of safety in our body, the experience can frighten and retraumatize us. Psychological techniques that attempt to blast through layers of protection to get to the root of the trauma often result in overwhelming clients and producing experiences that are difficult to integrate. There are no shortcuts to psychological healing or spiritual development. We can charge our way through the psyche only to spend decades integrating the healing, or we can seek wise and skillful direction and slowly practice, heal, mature, and transform.

Hastening the pace of psychological healing can even be an unconscious self-protective mechanism that works to stymie change or prevent us from fundamentally understanding ourselves. When I was in my twenties, I pursued every available method to excavate my psyche and exorcise the pain of my still-unnamed trauma once and for all. It took me several years to see this type of exertion as inefficient and oftentimes futile. I lacked the ego strength and preparedness to feel and integrate deeper levels of my experience, in addition to being without skillful therapeutic guidance to help me establish a workable pace of healing. Throughout this process, I fooled myself into thinking I was heroic, but I was actually not progressing any more than I was psychologically ready to.

Somatic inquiry and yoga practice work so well together because both support conscious entry into the body, albeit through different portals. Additionally, both teach us to pace our own opening. Experienced yoga practitioners often have an easier time learning to feel emotion as sensation within their bodies. Even if they haven't experienced the emotional level of the asanas, they have at least some familiarity with tolerating a variety of sensations in the body. When taught how to enter the emotional level of their body, therefore, they are able to follow the directions more readily.

At the same time, people can also use yoga as a buffer against feeling. Whereas the effort of "pushing though" in yoga practice may bring some benefit for a short while, this rarely works in psychotherapy. If yoga practitioners or teachers have experienced trauma, it can require abundant patience and skilled help to access the emotional level of the body, particularly when they have come to yoga to escape the trauma or attempt to transcend it. Even if we consider ourselves spiritually developed, it might take longer than expected to process and metabolize the emotional body. Accordingly, we need to respect our natural rhythms as well as those of the people we aspire to help. Trauma diagnosis and treatment differ from person to person. In the case of spiritually related traumas—for example, those caused by wounded or corrupt leaders—the treating clinician should have experience, familiarity, and an open mind with respect to spiritual practice. When it comes to yoga, for example, therapists need to help the client distinguish when the practice will serve as a highly effective treatment and when the client will employ it to avoid or subvert the healing process.

As the maxim goes, "Give someone a fish and you feed them for a day. Teach them *how* to fish and you feed them for a lifetime." Learning to feel emotion as sensation in the body is not easy to do, but the skill has benefits that can last a lifetime. I think it's one of the most important revelations of somatic practice as taught by both psychology and yoga. As mentioned in chapter 6, a friend of mine only began to feel her body when it was racked with cancer. The body is tremendously alive through and through, and for many people discovering the capacity to feel it from within is life-changing and precious. Ideally, we don't wait until we are dying to make this discovery.

Traumatic events that impact the body must necessarily involve the body in their healing. Unfortunately, the use of yoga and somatic methods for psychological healing is still not widely accepted in mainstream psychology, and only a handful of insurance companies and mental-health facilities recognize them as valuable tools for recovery and wellness. I hope this book plays a part in increasing that awareness.

HEALING TRAUMA THROUGH
EMOTIONALLY SENSITIVE YOGA

During my internship to become a licensed psychotherapist, I taught yoga to at-risk adolescent girls for two years. A number of these girls were gang members. On the first day of yoga class, girls from both the red and blue gangs gathered in my office and a leader from the red gang tried to take control. She pointed to two girls in the blue group and demanded that they leave the room.

I held my ground. "*You* can leave if you'd like," I reminded her, "but yoga goes way beyond whatever colors you're wearing. You have to choose to be here with everyone else who wants to be here. Otherwise, yoga won't help." Sadly, she left, hopefully to return to yoga or other healing modalities when she was ready. However, everyone else stayed after I gave them a short demonstration, and the girls caught a glimpse of what yoga could offer them. Over the months, I slowly guided them into an awareness of their physical, emotional, and subtle bodies through asanas, breathwork, and guided meditation. Eventually, the girls began to open up about their abuses at home and in their gangs, and several shared the insecurities and pressures that led them into gang life. A couple even expressed their ambivalence about being involved in a life that hurts and separates people. Without yoga to help them regulate their nervous systems and provide a context for their suffering, I strongly doubt I would have convinced a group of teens from conflicting gangs to express their vulnerabilities like that.

Yoga is a powerful tool for healing trauma. As cited elsewhere in this book, yoga has also been documented to significantly reduce the effects of stress, depression, anxiety, immunity and eating disorders, ADHD, schizophrenia, phobic behavior, and psychosomatic problems. Yoga boosts mood and well-being and increases attention span, self-esteem, and the capacity to self-soothe. It improves social and coping skills, ego strength, family relationships, sleep patterns, school performance, occupational functioning, and quality of life.[9] Again, these benefits occur even without integrating yoga with psychological techniques, somatic modalities, trauma treatment practices, and the wisdom of neuroscience.

As explored earlier in this chapter, some traumas occur at precognitive or preverbal moments in our lives. Some people feel the need to express and heal what happened to them, but they lack the memories, words, or concepts to explain it. Other people want relief beyond what drugs, alcohol, and overeating offer, but they may feel crippled with shame or are simply not ready to talk yet. Yoga practice—especially when it is trauma-informed—can circumvent all of this while beginning the process of somatic healing.

Yoga directly teaches people to unwind their nervous system from within their bodies. As I looked at in chapter 5, yoga increases heart-rate variability, which results in an improved capacity to regulate the arousal of one's nervous system. Yoga viscerally demonstrates that we can open up to difficult sensations, tolerate, release, or shift them, and even transform these sensations into pleasurable experiences. Because the residue of trauma resides in the body, learning to gently and gradually move toward contractions and stuck places within the muscle and fascia (as well as the emotions contained within them) eventually leads to healing psychosomatic pains we may lived with our entire lives.

Yoga is the practice that healed 90 percent of my own autoimmune disorder. As I discharged stuck patterns, prana released itself throughout my body like an invisible but palpable medicine that brought healing energy where it was needed. This improved the quality of my breath, helped me notice and embody areas of numbness, and dramatically increased my energy and vitality.

As we learn more about yoga's benefits for working with emotions and healing trauma, more schools and brands of yoga are emerging with particular gifts and insights. Psychologists and yoga teachers such as David Emerson, Bo Forbes, Richard Miller, and Amy Weintraub have made important contributions to this growing field. Most schools share an emphasis on yoga's capacity to elicit and heal emotional and even traumatic material in the body, whether fostering opportunities to do so or meeting them spontaneously during practice. These approaches ideally help teachers and practitioners become familiar with the signs of strong arousal, methods to calm and modulate the nervous system, ways to unwind emotions through the body, and awareness into how practices can be misused or those that are contraindicated.

The approaches also differ quite a bit. Some schools of trauma and emotionally sensitive yoga suggest specific practices for addressing certain emotions and psychological conditions (anxiety, depression, insomnia, etc.) and trauma. Others teach practitioners to understand how the currents of emotion and trauma arise within them and how to discover "from the inside out" the optimal way to use yogic practices to address the individual's unique set of psychological challenges. The former approach is more formulaic, particularly helpful to populations and individuals who have little yoga experience, and it's usually drawn from the teacher's significant experience with practices that have been shown to address specific ailments. The latter method teaches students the skills and perspectives that allow them to let their bodies perceive which postures and practices they need to unwind and psychologically heal. I believe there is value in both approaches.

The trainings I lead tend to follow the second method of healing. My experience over the years has encouraged me to teach others the perspectives and techniques to allow them to enter and refine their own capacity to heal themselves and divine their own dreams. The maxim "One person's poison is another's medicine" is especially true when it comes to yoga, and I strongly believe in empowering others to discover their own medicine. The techniques presented in the following chapter reflect this conviction. To this end, I include psychoeducation in my trainings; students learn to understand and treat whatever layer of psychological ailment they are working with. This includes the following variables:

- how to create safe emotional space in oneself and in the classroom

- how to pay attention to the mood we create

- ways to attune to the emotional aspects of poses and practices

- how long to practice different poses

- what degree to lean into and back out of the poses

- how to maximize emotional healing and minimize the possibility of using yoga to buffer or reify psychological defenses and traumatic experience

Still another aspect of yoga's capacity to work with sympathetic and parasympathetic arousal comes from the benefits of practicing within a group. Even if we feel isolated, we are not. In the yoga classroom, our nervous systems attune to the environment around us, even if we are not aware of it. Those who have experienced trauma are often more sensitive to their environment due to the physiological remnants of the survival response (the need to be ready to defend oneself at a moment's notice). As the teacher sets the space for the group to engage in the synchronized practice of concentration, breath, and movement (and perhaps chanting or meditative inquiry), a process of entrainment often arises in which the individual's inner rhythms begin to align with those of the other practitioners and with the external rhythm set by the practice. Many who engage in kirtan—chanting sacred names or mantras as a group—experience this as a shared nervous system with the capacity to attune to healing sound vibrations. As always, the psychological safety and boundaries established by those who guide the space strongly influence the quality of entrainment and healing.

I love teaching dedicated yoga teachers and practitioners about psychology. Although there's no substitute for years of study and practice, even small amounts of awareness and knowledge of psychology, somatics, and trauma help yogis address psychological ailments and trauma more skillfully. I strongly feel that a combination of yoga and neuroscience-informed somatic therapy is the optimal medicine for healing acute and everyday trauma. However, not everybody who practices yoga will engage with therapy, and vice versa. Because yoga is popular and less expensive than psychotherapy, people who aren't ready to enter therapy can first enter the doorway of healing their trauma through yoga. Yoga teachers who possess an awareness of trauma, therefore, are in the position to offer healing and life-changing guidance.

THE HEALING POWER OF LOVE AND PLEASURE

We can also approach somatic healing through the cultivation of pleasure, wholeness, and well-being. Furthermore, we can learn to experience these qualities at the level of sensation in the body. According to many, love itself is the most powerful medicine. Therefore, love is the balm for trauma and so many other ailments that assail the human psyche. In the ancient Indian epic poem the Ramayana, Princess Sita writes to her Guru and Lover, Lord Rama:

> Love is greater than hate
> Love is greater than fear
> Love is greater than doubt
> Love is greater than impatience
> Love is greater than despair
> Love is greater than anger
> Love is greater than any pain to body or mind
> Love defeats loneliness
> Love defeats pride
> Love defeats jealousy
> Love defeats the death of mother and father
> Blind love has seen me
> through every corner of hell
> And it is love alone
> that shall prevail[10]

After years of working as a psychotherapist, I'm convinced that at least half of the healing of the therapeutic process comes from cultivating what is pleasurable, right, and working about my clients. I think it's crucial that we recognize what's good in our life and discover wholeness and pleasure in our body. Acknowledging and nurturing what is healthy and intact in our psyches moves us toward fulfillment and well-being.

Far too often when we work with emotional healing we overly focus on what's broken and painful. Unfortunately, many therapists and psychological methods support this approach. Of course, we need to face our painful emotions and stories, and we must encounter our shame with compassion and openness, but our healing will be limited if that's all we do. Building self-love while dismantling trauma through yoga and psychology actually increases the effectiveness of recovery, and it is essential that we learn to experience pleasure and wholeness in our body. Psychologist Rick Hanson, PhD, often notes that the brain is like Velcro for negative experiences but like Teflon for positive ones. He also writes:

> Working with the mind and body to encourage the development of what's wholesome—and the uprooting of what's not—is central to every path of psychological and spiritual development. Even if practice is a matter of "removing the obscurations" to true nature—to borrow a phrase from Tibetan Buddhism—the clearing of these is a progressive process of training, purification, and transformation. Paradoxically, it takes time to become what we already are. In either case, these changes in the mind—uncovering inherent purity and cultivating wholesome qualities—reflect changes in the brain. By understanding better how the brain works and changes—how it gets emotionally hijacked or settles into calm virtue, how it creates distractibility or fosters mindful attention, how it makes harmful choices or wise ones—you can take more control of your brain and therefore your mind.[11]

People who suffer from sexual trauma require healing that involves rediscovering sexual pleasure in the body. Doing so acts as a profound catalyst to help them release shame, traumatic memories, and emotions locked up in the body. Additionally, when skillfully explored in a tantric context (as described in chapter 6), sexual healing can lead to valuable spiritual experiences. In the right context, ecstasy acts as potent medicine for all forms of trauma—sexual, everyday, and developmental (namely, that experienced by those who were not modeled healthy sexuality when they were younger).

Yoga teaches that prana follows attention. Life force flows wherever we focus. We can remember this dictate during our healing process and learn to place sufficient attention on our wounding without over-emphasizing it. Through the complementary practices of yoga and psychology, we can skillfully balance our awareness between what still causes pain and what is already healed and whole.

"Fear can stop you loving," sings the English band Morcheeba. "Love can stop your fear." Fear can prove incredibly difficult to feel and work with, whether it arises as anxiety, panic, distress, or terror. In the body, fear is cold and uncomfortable, often manifesting as bracing or physical contraction. Fear haunts us throughout our life, often hiding behind other emotions like sadness and anger. Even when we attempt to address fear directly in a safe, therapeutic context, it quickly hides under thoughts, interpretations, and almost anything to keep us from the difficult work of feeling it.

When it comes to trauma, the best medicine is love. Psychological wounds, knots, and contractions—even the psyche itself—respond much more effectively to love than they do to force or judgment. In this regard, self-love is not frivolous or indulgent, but actually necessary to heal trauma. Incredible healing comes when we combine mindfulness with self-compassion, and when we practice yoga well, it is a direct, embodied form of self-love. Self-soothing is one way we can use love as a remedy to fear. Kind words, embracing our own body, a gentle voice, a warm bath, a walk in nature—opportunities to engage in soothing thoughts and actions are all around us. For years I wore soft fabrics and velvet shirts just so that I'd be more inclined to rub my arms and embrace myself.

When I teach psychologically informed asana classes, I begin with different versions of Mountain Pose (*Tadasana*), which yoga classes often start with. Instead of holding hands in prayer in front of their chests, I ask people to explore the pose with their arms in a self-hugging position or with their hands resting gently on their belly. Even simple changes like this can create a stable, loving, and self-soothing atmosphere in relationship to our body.

THE GIFTS OF TRAUMA

Most people who have been traumatized are surprised to learn that their trauma can also be an asset. To be specific, the more we face our trauma, the more wisdom, transformation, and opening we gain. If we pay attention to trauma and the gifts it brings, the gifts have a chance to flourish in us. Here are four such gifts that yoga and psychotherapy can help to transform.

1. **Empathy**   If we can keep our hearts open even as they are breaking, we become better able to feel and connect with others and their suffering. People who have suffered from trauma can often access great empathy for the suffering of others. With the requisite training and inner work, psychotherapists and yoga teachers who have experienced trauma can learn to establish and maintain healthy boundaries with clients, which will actually allow them to activate their empathy and become more permeable without getting overwhelmed by others' suffering. This balance is crucial to prevent overwhelm and additional wounding.

2. **Sensitivity**   Understandably, people who have experienced sympathetic/hyperarousal symptoms for much of their lives tend to be hypersensitive. With yoga and psychological inquiry, hypersensitivity transforms into energetic awareness. This can feel psychic at times, but it's actually quite natural, like the phenomenon of receiving a phone call from a friend you were just thinking about. Someone with heightened sensitivity has the ability to attune to the

energy of others and the physical space they share. Like empathy, this level of sensitivity empowers our ability to connect. Working through trauma allows us to harness this unique gift and benefit anyone we choose to encounter.

3. **Spiritual Transformation**   Trauma often breaks people open at an early age. It leaves them with fundamental questions about love, connection, suffering, the meaning of life, healing, and service. In this way, trauma opens our hearts to spiritual longing. My teacher Lee Lozowick wrote a wonderful prayer: "Please give me a wound of love that only God can heal." Trauma can leave us feeling overly porous, but this permeability can offer us more doorways into our own embodiment as well as the mystical states offered in yoga and meditation. Again, committing to the necessary inner work enables us to access this profound gift of trauma without succumbing to the popular pitfall of spiritual bypassing.

4. **Healing**   So many of our greatest teachers and leaders have experienced some type of trauma in their lives. It actually seems rare to me that people enter the path of yoga or psychological inquiry with a healthy, intact, and supportive childhood. Accordingly, the commitment to our own healing allows us to offer the same to others. Countless people come to yoga through extreme circumstances such as chronic illness, accidents, severe injuries, and addictions. Yoga can be incredibly powerful medicine in this way, and it enables these people to communicate yoga's potential when they themselves become teachers. The wounded healer is such an important archetype for our time, and it's paramount that those who suffer trauma understand that recovery and empowerment are possible. As Peter Levine writes, "Trauma is a fact of life. It does not, however, have to be a life sentence."[12]

OUR SHARED EMOTIONAL INTENSITY

In 2006, I attended the Kagyu Monlam, a great gathering at the Bodhi Tree in Bodh Gaya, India, where the Buddha is said to have attained enlightenment. My body was severely weakened and tormented by the intestinal aches that come from "Delhi belly" when the Seventeenth Gyalwang Karmapa—the head of the Kagyu lineage of Tibetan Buddhism—addressed the thousands of monastics and others who had gathered. The Karmapa began, "The greatest challenge you will experience as monks and nuns . . ."

Despite the pain, I sat up in rapt attention. What was he going to tell them? Would it be about their struggles with celibacy, a life of endless service, waking up at four in the morning to bathe in freezing water and meditate, or endlessly scrubbing the monastery's floors? I had lived in an ashram, so I knew some of the sacrifices involved regarding austerities, discomforts, conflicts with others, and endless practice. But the Karmapa didn't talk about any of these things. He continued, ". . . is the challenge of dealing with your human emotions."

This is one of the most important teachings I have ever received. No matter who we are, no matter what our experience, every one of us has a complex and varied emotional life simply by virtue of being human. Similarly, we all share a need to articulate that emotional intensity, to strive toward happiness, and thrive. If we can turn toward this intensity and allow it to emerge with compassionate awareness, we can peel away the barriers that separate us from ourselves, others, and life itself. Doing so is a tremendous act of self-love, and it's one of the possibilities available to us when we integrate yoga and psychology.

PART III

METHODS, TOOLS, AND PRACTICES

8

THE YOGA & PSYCHE
METHOD TOOLBOX

May the heat of suffering become the fire of love.[1]
LEE LOZOWICK

Now that we've delved into the ways that yoga and psychology conjoin and intersect, it's time to apply their integrated practices to our own lives. The Yoga Sutras teach that "practice implies repetition." Ideally, this means that we explore these practices throughout our day whether we find ourselves in a psychotherapy session, holding a particular asana, teaching a group of students, or spending time with our children. Remembering to engage these practices for short periods throughout the day—even thirty seconds to two minutes at a time—will bring profound benefit to your life.

Although much of this book addresses the work of yoga teachers, therapists, and mental-health workers, the material applies to a wide range of disciplines and environments, so I encourage you to explore these practices in your own areas of expertise. When you begin to teach and share this material with others, be sure that you feel well-prepared and have practiced with the techniques. At the same time, I encourage you to risk, stretch into new places, make mistakes, and own and take responsibility for what you do know and understand. Remember that all of us are on some part of a learning curve that never ends—we'll never run out of opportunities to grow and integrate.

Before we get into the different practices and the Ten-Step Yoga & Psyche Method, I want to offer three overriding principles to consider: creating psychological safety, discernments for bringing somatics and yoga into the therapy room, and discernments for working somatically in the yoga room.

CREATING PSYCHOLOGICAL SAFETY

Psychological safety refers to an invisible yet tangible sense we communicate to students and clients. It lets them know that we welcome their experience, that we encourage them to make their own discoveries, that we will hold confidential space for them while they do so, and that we will not get overwhelmed by their experience.

Ideally, we become someone who can offer psychological safety by knowing our own psyche intimately. We do this by engaging our own psychological inquiry over an extended period of time—maybe just a few years at the outset, but reengaging the process throughout our lives, particularly during major transitions and stages of development. The space we offer others directly depends on the depth of our own exploration. Clients and yoga students feel the level of psychological safety in the room, and we express this directly through our experience, as well as through skillful use of language.

That being said, it's essential to tell clients and students that whatever exchange happens is confidential. In a group, asking students to nod if they understand and agree to confidentiality will immediately heighten a sense of psychological safety in the room. It's also important to remind them that trust and safety don't come right away—they are organically built through time and experience. Clients and students should feel free to share at their own pace, and as much or as little as they feel safe doing so. Furthermore, they should know the value of monitoring this sense of safety for themselves.

As mentioned, clients and students also attain a sense of safety when they experience that their powerful feelings—even when expressed through tears, shaking, and anger—can be held by someone who isn't overpowered by their intensity. I recommend beginning your relationship with clients or students by letting them know directly that their feelings are welcome. In the yoga room, tell the class that you won't question these emotions—sorrow, happiness, fear, bliss, anxiety, or anything else—unless they ask for your support, and let them know that they are welcome to continue whatever practice they are doing (or back off) in order to intensify or diminish the power of the emotion. As a therapist or yoga teacher, you may feel this agreement to be tacit or understood, but verbalizing it speaks to the unconscious mind and conveys explicit permission for students to explore their inner intensity. When you articulate this invitation, it brings their attention to the psychological level of their experience—in yogic philosophy, this is called the *manomaya kosha*. Simply being aware of the emotional aspect of our experience helps us to integrate it with our yoga practice or experience of therapy.

Regarding yoga, it's perfectly legitimate to create a space that does not focus on the psychological and emotional levels of experience, but you should be clear about what you want to offer as a teacher (and, if you're a student, what you are looking for in a teacher). However, creating a space of psychological safety in the yoga room allows students to process psychological material through the practice. It helps them move gently through their unconscious obstacles and into subtler levels of their experience and well-being; in addition, it offers the various physical and spiritual benefits for which yoga is well known.

DISCERNMENTS FOR BRINGING SOMATICS AND YOGA INTO THE THERAPY ROOM

I want to mention four important variables here for those who want to include somatic psychology and gentle yoga practices in the psychotherapeutic context:

Be well trained. It's incredibly important to receive significant training in some form of well-developed somatic therapy and yoga before bringing it to clients. We store everything—especially trauma—in our bodies, and opening up can release powerful emotions and physical responses. The therapist should know how to keep clients from becoming overwhelmed or retraumatized and should be able to steer them toward progressive healing and integration.

Timing is everything.   Through experience, therapists learn how to pace yogic and somatic interventions, specifically how long to focus on them before backing out and integrating. Usually, this means slowing down and focusing on basic interventions rather than sophisticated techniques.

Clients might not feel ready to bring or interested in bringing yogic or somatic practices into their therapy, particularly if they are just beginning or are in crisis. People with no previous therapeutic experience often come to therapy with a strong need to download their stories, secrets, shame, trauma, and deep pain, or they express an immediate need to manage a particular predicament in their life. Some clients just need to feel listened to, empathized with, and have their feelings—rage, jealousy, fear, and so on—normalized. An alarming number of people come to therapy believing that they are far more messed up than other people are, and they find tremendous healing in discovering that they are simply "normal neurotics." It's important to build trust and not rush this fundamental work.

Ideally, when I bring up the idea of doing somatic practices and a client doesn't feel ready, they tell me as much. However, sometimes clients don't have the language to do this, or else any number of other factors—their projections onto me, their wish to be a good client, their desire to heal quickly—can prevent them from trusting their own instinct to go slowly. When I bring in somatic practices too early, my attempts either fall flat or they aren't as effective as they would be if the client were more ready. When I recognize this, I let the client know that it seems like the timing isn't right for these practices, and I suggest we revisit them down the road—perhaps between three and six months later. Needless to say, when they don't take to somatic or yoga practices right away (or ever), it's important that the client doesn't feel ashamed or that they have failed in some way.

Ease into the practice.   Clients who practice yoga or other forms of spiritual work sometimes come to therapy eager to work with somatics or yoga. For some people, this eagerness is more intellectual than embodied. Other clients carry wounds they have never faced, or they feel afraid about opening up to what's stored in their body. For these reasons, it's crucial to ease into these practices and help the client regulate their own pacing (see the sections on titration and pendulation later in this chapter). It's fine to begin with simple practices and keep doing them for a long time. People connect with certain aspects of practice more than others, and there's no need to try to speed through any somatic or yogic work. Easing into the practice is part of the practice itself. There's no rush, and nowhere to go, really. Instead, encourage the clients to focus on their experience of the practices and whatever ongoing insights and benefits they receive.

Less is more.   Some of the somatic tools seem quite simple, but they are actually potent practices. Accordingly, we need to use these tools wisely and avoid pushing too hard, reliving painful experiences, and retraumatizing ourselves or others. Far too many approaches emphasize catharsis in the healing process when people actually need to experience smaller, more sustainable, and progressive changes.

As I mentioned in the last chapter, I once facilitated groups for Latina at-risk teens, many of whom were gang members. I was studying a lot about trauma at the time. Excited by my new storehouse of sophisticated tools, I often tried to employ complex techniques to work with the girls in their crises and predicaments. More often than not, my interventions were met with blank faces and silence. However, when I shared the most basic somatic tools of resourcing and learning to feel and create safety inside their body—in addition to simple yoga and meditation practices—the girls blossomed. One day, I asked them to visualize a light of whatever color they desired in the shape of an egg inside the center of their hearts. Then I asked them to imagine slowly placing themselves inside that egg. I let the girls know that we would only be doing this practice for one minute, and that if at any time they felt dissociated or uncomfortable that they could simply open their eyes and look to me for reassurance. Each week we added an additional minute to the practice. After just a few weeks, one of the young women reported that she had never felt safe in her life before doing this practice. Another was amazed to discover that she could create a safe place inside her own body even if the world around her felt dangerous or threatening.

This is just to say that simple practices can go a long way. "Slow is the new fast," declared one of my students after exploring these techniques herself. We don't need sophisticated techniques when straightforward exercises (with proper timing) will yield equally profound results.

DISCERNMENTS FOR WORKING SOMATICALLY IN THE YOGA ROOM

Here are some key points of discernment for practitioners and teachers of yoga. There's some overlap here with the variables presented in the previous section, but please note how these refer specifically to the yoga studio. Let's start with discernments for yoga practitioners first. Even if you are attending a class with a teacher who isn't somatically trained—or maybe you're doing yoga in dyad practice with others, at home alone, or somewhere else by yourself—you can apply these principles and practices.

Slow down.   No matter where you are, it's important to control the pace of your practice without feeling pushed or corrected. Slow down to give yourself the space to explore the psychological levels of your experience. How much you need to slow down changes over time and depends on the practice as well as your level of energy or stress. It also depends on what comes up psychologically in your body. When you physically strain yourself in a pose, you have less attention to explore the psychological level of your experience. The more you do a practice, of course, the easier it is to attune to all aspects of your experience, even while engaging strenuously.

Listen to your body.   After you've learned the basic structure of a pose and can execute it safely, you can listen to your body to discover adjustments from within. Once you have learned to tune in to the psychological level of your experience during yoga, your body gives you cues and clues to progressively release and process your emotions through small, internal self-adjustments. Some of these may be physical—slowing down your breath, for example—but others might take the form of softening your attitude or changing the voice you use to speak to yourself. When you access your body's inner wisdom in this way, you can begin to slowly explore how it can teach you to heal yourself on various levels from the inside out.

Inquire, but compassionately. Speak nicely to yourself as you explore the emotional and somatic levels of your experience and bring them into your awareness during yoga practice. Use a sweet, kind, gentle, and understanding voice as you talk to yourself—even if it feels like you're faking it. As you work with the practices given below, compassionately check in with your feelings—are you mad, sad, glad, or scared? Pay attention to different parts of your body and gently explore the sensations and emotions that are held there.

Ideally, our inner voice becomes softer over time—more self-loving and life-affirming. This in itself is a tremendous psychological break-through, despite whatever challenges we continue to face. Our inquiry becomes more about learning to "love the questions themselves," as poet Rainer Maria Rilke urges, than it is about discovering finite answers. As you explore your emotions during asana practice, your body processes feelings as they arise, yet you continue to receive the physical and spiritual benefits of yoga. When I practice in this way, I feel like I'm getting a "three-for-one" deal: a cleansing workout for my body, a boost for my spirit, and a helpful self-therapy session to integrate whatever comes up in my life and body.

Now let's look at some guidelines for those of us who also teach yoga:

Be well trained. I talked about this earlier in a different context, but it bears repeating here. It's crucial to get some solid somatic training before teaching these practices in your yoga class. Somatics has become a buzzword in yoga studios and among yoga teachers in the United States and increasingly throughout the world. Because discovering the inner world of the psychological body and deep psyche can feel so revelatory and exciting, teachers often want to jump in and teach somatics right away. That's wonderful. However, teachers need to keep in mind that when we open the body—ours or those of our students—we open to whatever trauma is contained within the body. So it's wise to ground ourselves with solid guidance and prepare to receive whatever comes up so that we don't risk becoming overwhelmed, and can guide our students skillfully. It's also important to understand our own scope of practice and knowledge—we should discern when and where to refer people for further help. I also recommend exploring somatic material as a client—preferably for two or three years—before beginning to teach it. There are no shortcuts to this work, and no matter what you say in the yoga room, students will intuit the results of your own psychological work. Furthermore, they will unconsciously sense "permission" from you to feel more or less intensely depending on the inner work you have done.

Begin with safer practices.　When teaching, always begin with safer practices, like resourcing or learning to feel emotion as sensation in the body. You don't get enough depth or continuity of contact with students in short, weekly classes to engage the more sophisticated somatic techniques; this instead tends to happen when you're working in a more intensive context, such as an immersion, weekend program, or ongoing group. The practices taught in this chapter are each powerful and complete within themselves. You can also progressively layer them on each other and work with each of them over a long period of time. I have personally found no endpoint when applying these practices to my own (or my clients') processes. Simply helping your students attune to the emotional level of their experience during asana, and learning to feel their emotions as sensations in their body during yoga practice, can itself be life changing.

Use skillful language. The words we speak can invite students into their own embodied emotional and somatic experience. Having worked my way through graduate school as a massage therapist, I was surprised in my studies of trauma and somatics to discover that you can guide people into their inner body without using physical touch. Educate your students by letting them know that they can experience any and all emotions as physical sensation in their bodies, which is also where the emotions are processed. Teach them that it is possible to learn to use their yoga practice not only for physical and spiritual benefits, but also for psychological ones.

Create an invitation. In your own words, let your students know that you welcome their emotional experience in the room. Tell them that they are free to feel whatever arises as they practice, and that if they need to take a break, cry, shake, or pause, they should trust and follow this impulse. Remind them that you will not question or judge them. Again, it might be apparent to you that you are fine with whatever students are experiencing, but they often don't know unless you tell them. Some of my clients in psychotherapy who also practice yoga have said that they have wanted to cry in class or just stop and feel an emotion intensely, but they felt too inhibited to do so, or they feared that the teacher would judge them—even if they suspected this was probably not the case. For this reason, we need to invite students to allow their emotional experience into the yoga room, and we should repeat this invitation regularly.

However, you should only extend this invitation if you feel confident in your ability and readiness to follow through. I've worked with several yoga teachers who don't know how to respond when students express powerful emotions, or they become confused about helpful, ethical boundaries. Teachers can optimize their use of somatic practices by exploring their own body and mind in a meaningful, ongoing way.

INTEGRATED PRACTICES

With the above three principles established, I want to offer six fundamental practices chosen for their accessibility, practicality, and effectiveness. These practices come out of my long and sincere inquiry into these subjects, my study of Peter Levine's Somatic Experiencing method, and from my experience teaching yoga and somatic practices to students of all types around the world.

Practice 1: Learning to Feel Emotion in the Body

We can experience all emotion as sensation in the body, and learning to do so is often a turning point in one's inner healing. I'm including a list of "feeling" words for bodily sensations below; this list was created by the Somatic Experiencing Trauma Institute.[2]

When you read these words out loud for clients or students, suggest that they gently scan their body to note the presence and location of these feelings. Simply identifying the sensations of emotions in the body—and bringing compassionate awareness to them—immediately enables us to process, heal, and integrate emotions on a somatic level. These words can also be used as suggestions and options to support clients to learn to identify the sensations they experience in their body as they process emotional material. In no particular order, these possible bodily sensations include:

Hot/warm	Cold
Slow	Fast
Loose	Stuck
Relaxing	Empty
Tingly	Floating
Tight	Calm
Shaky	Flowing
Constricted	Front/back
Moving Up/Down	Dizzy
Numb	Buzzing
Opening	Itching
Burning	Tension
Lightness	

The questions "How do you feel?" and "Where do you feel what you feel in your body?" may seem novel and sometimes unsettling to people who find it difficult to detect or describe how they feel at any given time. People might be able to identify particularly strong emotions such as sorrow, heartbreak, or rage; they may even be able to connect these to their heart or gut. However, a surprising number of people have difficulty identifying even the most potent of feelings, let alone the vast array of emotions that lie along the spectrum of pleasure and pain. It can be a life-changing revelation to discover that we experience *all* emotion as sensation in the body and subsequently to learn to process emotions through somatic awareness. Thomas Hanna described somatics as referring to "the body as perceived from within the first-person perception . . . the human being as experienced by himself [or herself] from the inside."[3] For some people, this reentry into the body is felt as a spiritual experience and process.

With safety and skill, we can learn to enter the body slowly, lovingly, and progressively—gently turning toward emotions and even traumatic experiences that we have feared or avoided feeling our whole lives, and transforming them into authentic gifts. We discern for ourselves that we can experience even powerful emotions as sensations in the body that are always moving and changing. Some of these may feel unpleasant or uncomfortable, especially at first. However, as we become more familiar with the practice and meet our sensations with awareness and compassion, they typically transform into something else. Noticing this, we gain the courage and curiosity to face our emotions, feel them in our bodies, and witness how tensions, patterns, memories, and emotions gradually metabolize and release.

Here's a loose outline for the practice:

1. To begin, take a few slow, deep, and natural (that is, not forced) breaths. If you feel any tensions in your body, try to release them.

2. Next, bring your awareness to everything in your body below your neck, scanning slowly to sense what you are feeling in the various areas of your body.

3. As you continue to breathe and pay attention to different areas of your body that hold tension, emotion, memories, and images, use your breath and movement to release them. If you are engaging this practice while in asana, allow your body to gently adjust your posture in order to unwind and process emotion in any way it naturally wants to. Simply bringing compassionate attention and breath to emotions as they live inside the body will enable them to change and gently unwind, just as the body does during asana. In addition to yoga practice, this is a process you can integrate into talk therapy, self-inquiry, or dyad practice.

4. You can also explore the following questions when engaging in this practice:

- What do you feel in your body?

- Where do you feel the emotion?

- What else do you notice as you feel that sensation?

- How would you describe its shape, size, or color?

- Does the feeling spread?

- What is its temperature and texture?

- What are the images or memories that come with it?

- Where are the borders and boundaries of the sensation, and where do you stop feeling it? (For example: top, bottom, front, back.)

- Where does the sensation change into something else?

- How would you describe these boundaries of sensation?

- Does it stay the same or change as you pay attention to it?

- When you stay with what you are feeling, what happens next?

These simple questions yield deeper and more nuanced responses from within ourselves when practiced over time. They can also transform the way we process our emotions on a daily basis. When I refer to *processing* trauma and emotion, I hope it's clear that I don't mean that they go away forever. They are part and parcel of life itself. *Processing* in this context means that we move through our feelings and experiences more quickly, with more ease, and with far less fear. When we turn toward emotions and memories and connect them with bodily sensations, we viscerally come to understand that remembering past events, trauma, and painful memories does not necessarily need to be overwhelming. We can actually find the experience to be freeing and healing.

As we explore this practice further, we discover that emotions are not simply sensations—they are comprised of continually moving, changing, and layered sensate experiences. For example, we might initially connect feelings of anger to tightness in the belly, but further exploration reveals that our belly entails multiple layers and dimensions—a front and back, sides, and perhaps a sense of blurriness as to where it ends and other parts of the body begin. As we explore the details of our sensations, we might also discover that forgotten memories, new emotions, or novel visions and insights appear. What we perceive as *inside* and *outside* the body may begin to change or merge. Accordingly, our connection to the natural world may also change.

As we learn to move our awareness throughout the body, we might be surprised to find areas that are more difficult to feel—even numb—whereas other areas offer more sensation and movement. Perhaps some are even blissful. Sometimes areas of our body that contain intense pain also offer deep pleasure. As we continue to explore emotion as sensation, new levels of long-held tension and trauma unwind and release from within, and we are progressively liberated at deeper levels of psychological experience and somatic tension.

Although we may be accustomed to feeling certain emotions in specific areas of the body (sadness in the heart, anger in the belly), it's best not to assume that we will perceive a given emotion in the same place or way as we did previously—or even as others might commonly experience it. Trauma and the emotional life of the body are complex, layered, and ever changing. We gain more benefit by exploring emotion in the body freshly each time we turn toward it, allowing ourselves to gain the greatest amount of information and to process our experience more efficiently. We begin to experience more confidence, joy, self-esteem, and pleasure in our bodies as pain and trauma release. We also learn to move through life with the empowered awareness that we are actually capable of processing emotions in our bodies.

Practice 2: Tracking Sensation in the Body (and in Others' Bodies)

We pay close attention to sensations as they move through the body, allowing them to do so and noting any images, memories, and emotions that arise with them. As we track ourselves in this way, we discover that sensations can move, metabolize, and transform rather quickly when we bring loving, compassionate, and nonjudgmental awareness to them. We find ourselves getting stuck in our lives less often because we can process emotion in our bodies, and when we do get stuck, we remember that tracking the sensations of stuckness in the body allows us to get unstuck more quickly.

Once we are able to track sensations in our own bodies, we can begin to track the sensations of others. Therapists and teachers can use this powerful tool to empathize with others at a somatic level while maintaining boundaries and not taking on the pain of others in an unhealthy way. Here's an outline to the practice of attending to the physical sensations of others:

1. Drop your awareness into your body and scan the area beneath your neck. Bring your arms, legs, belly, heart, and the rest of your body into awareness.

2. Choose to set your personal experience to the side for now and bring your attention to the person in front of you (client, student, dyad partner, etc.).

3. Note the person's posture, the patterns of their breathing, gestures, or any other somatic sensations that are visible, and sense what these might feel like in your own body.

4. As you guide the person toward exploring emotion as sensation in their body, feel your own body in the noted areas and allow yourself to taste or sense what they are experiencing. Gently feel into those same sensations, breathing patterns, gestures, or postures in your own body. (You can work with not getting overwhelmed or taking on your clients' feelings by using the practice of "titration" later in this chapter.)

5. Watch for subtle signs of movement, holding, or release. Invite the person to articulate what they are perceiving.

6. As they articulate the experience, visualize whatever images they report and continue to allow yourself to feel their sensations in your own body.

7. As the person shifts in their body, follow the movement in your own body.

8. Always support the client by ending a session in a somatically and emotionally grounded place (see the next section on resourcing). Gently guide the client back to this reference in their bodies, and also allow yourself to return to a centered place in your own body.

As therapists, we benefit from this practice by learning to put our own experience aside and allowing ourselves to somatically feel another person's experience, and we practice doing so in a way that provides safe and healthy boundaries while simultaneously expressing our care. When we feel others in this way, it expands our capacity for empathy. The client or yoga student experiences this viscerally, thereby receiving tremendous support. For even short periods of time, they feel in their body that someone else holds their experience with them and that they are not alone with it. In tracking others' emotions as sensations in our own body, and by discovering a way to feel deeply with the other person without getting overwhelmed, we discover that we as human beings share a number of common emotions. In this way, all of us feel less alone and more connected with others, reminded that we all have a vulnerable and profound core in common.

Practice 3: Resourcing

Even though this is a straightforward practice, people regularly tell me that it's the most powerful somatic tool they've learned to use. In short, resourcing teaches us to consciously allow or invoke pleasure, safety, wholeness, fullness, sensuality, sexuality, joy, and well-being in the body. For those who have experienced and suffered intense trauma, resourcing often restores a sense of basic okayness that they may have lost. I've found that learning to establish pleasure and safety in the body is often more healing than what we gain by revisiting trauma. When we learn to create a climate of inner safety, the petals of our psyche organically unfold one by one. Old wounds dissipate more easily in an inner climate of increasing pleasure and self-love. Our psyche just needs small gestures of consistent nourishing and safe spaces in which to unfold.

Everyone possesses resources. Resources take the form of anything (or anyone) that supports and nurtures a sense of physical, emotional, mental, or spiritual well-being. Resources can be internal, external, or both. When trauma occurs, instinctive resources for protection and self-defense can become overwhelmed. Developing inner resources can help balance the nervous system and serve as a source of strength and support; it can also provide us with a sense of calm and wholeness, even in the face of uncertainty and difficulty.

Psychology, trauma-healing methods, and somatics have developed powerful tools for resourcing. Yoga offers an additional wellspring, including asanas, sequences, visualizations, breath practices, mantras, and community in addition to the perspectives offered by the philosophical aspects of yoga. Learning to utilize resources through various means empowers us to become emotionally flexible and capable of adjusting to life's intensities with more ease and grace. Remember that prana follows attention. Resourcing allows us to learn to be present with experiences such as spaciousness, wholeness, and the goodness in our lives, and it helps us enjoy them. When we have been traumatized, we often have to learn to tolerate pleasure in small doses, for even though we may long for joy, the feel of it can prove strange and unusual. It takes practice to trust that it is safe to allow ourselves to feel pleasure, wholeness, and goodness in our bodies. Here are five ways to explore resourcing for yourself and others:

1. **Resourcing through the Body**   You can engage this type of resourcing in seated meditation practice or during psychological inquiry in dyads or with a therapist. Begin by taking a few slow, deep breaths, and relax any surface tension when you exhale. As you bring awareness to your body at the emotional/psychological level of sensations, notice which areas feel more active and energized and in which places you feel less present, or even numb. Ask questions to help you or others explore places of wellness and pleasure in your body. Try these:

   - Can you find any sense (small or large) of wellness, wholeness, safety, pleasure, or spaciousness anywhere in your body? If so, where is it?

   - What do the front, back, sides, and boundaries of that pleasure (or spaciousness, wholeness, etc.) feel like?

   - What are the colors, associated images, or memories that it brings with it?

   - How would you describe its temperature? Is it warm or cold?

   - As you stay with the pleasure (or spaciousness, wholeness, etc.), does it stay the same or change?

Begin to explore pleasure by gently extending and exploring these sensations, really taking the time to discover what positive emotion and enjoyment feel like at the level of sensation. Acknowledge to yourself and students or clients that it can take some time—and significant patience—for many to learn to feel a sense of pleasure and wholeness in our bodies, particularly if we were never taught or modeled how to experience such things or if we have been traumatized.

2. **Resourcing through Nature Imagery**   In this form of resourcing, we, a partner, or client come up with an image from nature that inspires nourishment, pleasure, safety, relaxation, and well-being. This can take the form of a place we've been to—perhaps a special beach or by a favorite tree—or it can be entirely imagined. As this image comes to mind, explore it with questions similar to those in the list above (e.g., "What is the temperature?" and "Are you alone or with others?" and "What textures surround you?"). While feeling into your body, place awareness on the colors, setting, temperature, wind, sun, and quality of the air in this beautiful place.

Next, hold that nature image in your mind as you drop awareness into your body—anywhere beneath your neck, lightly scanning your body to notice areas of heightened awareness or numbness. Allow the nature image to transpose itself onto your body, and investigate how you can experience that superimposition as sensation in your body. Following this practice is like engaging asanas with our emotions, and just like physical asanas, we learn and refine it through practice. Some people report being able to calm their nervous system easily, even when they first engage in this practice, whereas others require more patience.

For those who don't feel pleasure or wholeness when they sense into their bodies, invoking nature imagery serves as an accessible way to begin to do so. Because we encounter the imagery as something neutral, we more readily connect with the psychological safety and space needed to allow more pleasure and wholeness into our experience. And as we gently and repeatedly bring our awareness back to the nurturing nature image as the mind wanders, we learn to stay with a sense of well-being and allow that experience to be sustained for longer periods of time. With repeated practice, we gradually remodel our nervous system toward well-being and wholeness.

A final note on this practice: It's important that the practitioner not use a place in nature they escaped to as a child. A nature image of this type often carries with it the memory of the trauma that brought the person to seek it out in the first place, so using the same location is not as effective when it comes to developing new structures for safety and pleasure within our bodies. Additionally, people raised in cities for most of their lives may not associate nature imagery with nourishment and safety—they might even feel scared or intimidated by nature. These people will experience better results by relying on the other approaches to resourcing.

3. **Resourcing through Yogic Imagery**   Following the previous examples of resourcing, begin by visualizing an image of a yogic deity or archetype that you feel a connection to. If you are not familiar with specific deities, you can allow an image of a benevolent god or goddess to emerge in your awareness. As with nature resourcing, allow the image to be superimposed onto your own body, or if that is difficult, allow your awareness to move between the image and your own body. Begin to notice how the deity, or what it inspires, is felt as sensation and resourcefulness in your own body and allow the experience to expand and deepen using the previous inquiry questions to further explore the changing images, emotions, sensations, and insights as they emerge.

The Hindu pantheon abounds with imagery invoking the infinite qualities and aspects of the Divine. Yogic imagery speaks directly to the challenges and archetypes we face in life and offers us intricate maps along our journey to well-being. By resourcing these images, we can access a more universal sense of strength, faith, perseverance, beauty, and abundance. Although the wrathful deities found in Hindu and Buddhist iconography—for example Kali, Shiva, and the various forms of Mahakala—are ultimately beneficent, I recommend using imagery of kind, beautiful, and compassionate deities such as Lakshmi, Tara, Kuan Yin, or some version of the Earth Mother. People who aren't as familiar with these deities can use any benevolent image that comes to mind, even if it doesn't come with a specific name or familiar identity.

Sometimes learning this practice invokes mantras and prayers from traditions other than yoga. Spiritual practices that you were raised with or encountered throughout your life can offer new and surprisingly powerful resources. For example, a person might become reacquainted with, or newly encounter, the Hebrew Shemah chant, the tradition of chanting *Allah*, or speaking a line from a Christian prayer. When chanting aloud or reciting these words internally, we can bring our awareness to the emotional and somatic experience of our body and allow the sacred syllables and meanings to provide resourcing and to soften areas of holding and tension.

Resourcing through mystical imagery allows the possibility of new layers of insight, experience, and somatic integration to occur. And when we combine esoteric yogic practices with this type of resourcing, the results can be both psychological and spiritual.

4. **Resourcing through Asana**   To begin this physical type of resourcing, assume a nurturing and nondemanding yoga posture. Sink into the pose and use any props available to support more ease and comfort. Explore how you can become even more comfortable—and perhaps 5 percent kinder—toward yourself while in the pose, and see what you can release as you bring awareness to your body in this asana.

Check in with the tone of voice you use to speak to yourself. Turn toward yourself gently, asking how you are doing and letting your deep psyche know that you are here for yourself. Simply making the voice we address ourselves with in and out of yoga class more compassionate and loving can act as a tremendous resource.

If practicing in a dyad, one person can offer their hands to help the other adjust, soften, and feel more fully into the pose. Each partner takes a turn and learns to feel, request, and receive touch and safe physical support in the process of their own unwinding. Keep in mind that when we delve into the practices of titration and pendulation (explained next), this resourced asana becomes the place from which we enter and come out of somatic practice. Accordingly, explore these asanas extensively to discover their capacity to provide pleasure and support.

It's important to recognize that the asana one person considers a resource will not be so for someone else. In fact, one person's resource may be another's doorway into suffering, and this association can change for each of us from day to day. This is why we should allow people to identify their own resources through asana rather than transposing a series of poses designed to address everyone's proclivities and needs. It's best to begin fresh with each practice and inquiry in order to see how the emotional life of the body feels on any given day.

5. **Resourcing through Sun Salutations**   I once took a group of graduate students to study yoga in Varanasi, India. Every morning, we formed a silent procession to an outside platform just above the banks of the Ganges where it flowed through the city. As the sun rose, temple bells rang and thousands of people beneath us stood in the river or on its banks. They offered flowers and water, intoning the traditional Gayatri Mantra chanted at sunrise, high noon, and sunset. Additionally, they performed the series of

motions known as *Surya Namaskar* (Sun Salutation). After that profound experience, I began to include the Gayatri Mantra, supplications, prayers, and offerings to the way I practice and teach Sun Salutations, rather than simply the series of powerful, but not prayerful, set of asanas that I had understood Sun Salutations to be until then. Doing so has opened up an entirely new dimension of sun practice that others and I have experienced as profoundly nourishing and potently healing. At times we perceived, and witnessed others experience, that our bodies are actually prayers and can be used as such. I have repeated variations of this practice with students over the years and integrated it with other somatic exercises—for example, offering up one's sense of self-hatred or self-negation to the sun. The combination regularly brings people into beautiful experiences of embodied awareness.

To try this out yourself, chant or listen to the Gayatri Mantra as you begin the Surya Namaskar sequence. Contemplate its meaning and feel the vibration of the sound in your body as a prayer of alignment for the upper, middle, and lower layers of your consciousness. Ask for support to become connected and balanced with the rhythms of your body, the earth, and the cosmos. As you bend down in the forward folds of Sun Salutation, you bow to the sun as the giver of life. When you raise your arms back up, you scoop up the sacred waters of the world and offer it with flowers (and all of your imperfections) to the sun as a gift with gratitude. You can also offer that which no longer serves you—that is, what you wish to let go of in your life—as well as prayer and gratitude. Continue to bow, open your heart to the sun and light, and contemplate the sun and its life-giving properties as you move through the motions of Surya Namaskar and the Gayatri Mantra. For many of us, practicing in this way brings about an acute sense of psychological safety, well-being, peace, gratitude, and tremendous energy. You can turn this practice into a profound resource by using mantra, studying the practice more intensely, and continuing to explore the esoteric dimensions of Surya Namaskar.

Mantras—repeated words or phrases meant to invoke a divine name, universal principle, prayer, or intention—can serve as powerful inner resources. When I was engaged in intensive mantra practice as a young woman, I once found myself suddenly hydroplaning on a major highway near San Francisco at night. I watched as my car spun out of control toward the median, and an entire highway of traffic rushed straight at me. Having absolutely no control of the car, I remembered the mantra I had practiced with Yogi Ramsuratkumar in India and began to recite it. The next moment, the entire highway stopped, including my car and all others. I sat still in the rain, facing all of those vehicles stopped directly in front of me, with nobody harmed at all. I turned on my car, wheeled it around, and drove home. Although the near accident brought some shock and fear, the power of the mantra I had practiced to resource me was incredibly affirming, uplifting, and empowering. Similarly, I recommend the practice of kirtan as a potent form of yogic resourcing through mantra with the added benefit of community and the power of collective intention.

Practice 4: Titration

The word *titration* refers to the process of gradually applying a solution of a known concentration to a known volume of a different solution. In a yogic or somatic context, this means exploring a particular memory, wound, emotion, or contraction slowly, in small amounts, and for short periods of time by relying on an inner resource (for example, nature imagery or asana practice). We begin by invoking a sense of safety in the body through resourcing, and then we turn toward and titrate whatever it is we wish to explore. In titration we don't immediately feel into the center of a wound. Instead, we lightly touch its edge or outermost layer, ease into the emotion or trauma gradually, and feel and integrate it progressively at a sustainable pace.

Titration helps us realize that we have a choice about the manner in and depth to which we enter emotional states. We soon discover that we can make considerable strides by taking small steps toward our wounds, our shadow side, and the interior places that scare us, and then we can return to our inner resource. In the scientific principle of titration, one concentration is slowly added to another until the reaction reaches neutralization. In this context, the possibility exists to neutralize and defuse our contractions by engaging them within the body in digestible bits, all while relying on the safety of resourcing. Here's a brief guide to practicing titration in therapy, counseling, or dyad practice:

- Begin with one of the resourcing methods described earlier in this chapter.

- You can do this exercise with open or closed eyes, but closing the eyes often helps people feel into their bodies. However, if closing your eyes brings about dissociation or distraction, it's best to keep them open.

- Choose something you would like to work with: a certain pain, a physical or emotional contraction, a concern, or any type of challenge that comes to mind.

- Feel into the top layer of emotions and sensations that accompany this challenge in the body. The top layer can mean the top 5 percent, 3 percent, or less. I've had clients who prefer to feel into as little as the top .005 percent, and this also works.

- Try to stay with this experience for thirty to sixty seconds, and know that you are free to back out and return to a resourced place any time you begin to feel overwhelmed. Note: If you tell yourself, or a client, that you will be staying with the emotion for only thirty to sixty seconds, be sure not to stay there past that amount of time. Keeping within the stated time frame creates safety in our own psyche and that of our clients.

- If you're helping someone else with this practice, track their emotions and sensations in your own body as described above. Make sure that you don't become overwhelmed or shut down. Over time, your ability to support others in this way increases.

You can also explore titration in asana practice:

- Begin with an asana that provides a sense of resourcing.

- Now choose an asana to titrate that brings up resistance or some sort of physical or emotional challenge. However, don't pick a complex pose—you want to free up your awareness to the emotional aspect of your experience.

- Enter the pose as you normally might. Back out of the pose progressively to the degree that you can still access its physical and emotional imprint in a manageable way, beginning with 20 to 30 percent and even backing out as far as 90 percent.

- Now turn toward whatever sensations, emotions, memories, impressions, or images arise in your body. Feel and be with them for a short period of time—between fifteen and sixty seconds.

- Back out of this asana and return to the original resourced pose, or use some other resource.

- When applying titration to asana, you can also titrate between deeper and lesser intensity within the pose. For example, an ordinarily challenging pose can become resourced if titrated out of to a significant extent.

- If desired, repeat the above sequence between three and five times.

As you become familiar with using titration in asana, you discover that you can enter poses to greater or lesser degrees depending on the level of the pose you want to access. You learn how to use your yoga practice in various ways, including for psychological integration. At one point in your practice, you might choose to exert yourself physically to build muscle tone or work on your alignment, whereas at another point (or another posture) you may wish to slow down and process emotional content. At yet another point, you might explore the mystical aspect of the practice. In this way, titrating allows you to move fluidly through a practice and extract its various benefits—physical, psychological, and spiritual.

Practice 5: Pendulation

This practice refers to the process of moving between polarities in our experience—as if we were a pendulum. Pendulation occurs within us naturally unless we're disturbed by trauma or psychological wounding of some kind. We can, however, consciously discover pendulation by placing attention on the movement between polarities and opposites within us and bring these into relationship with each other. This practice helps create beneficial patterns in the nervous system that keep it from getting stuck in traumatic patterns, thereby slowly remodeling our brains. We can pendulate between feelings of joy, well-being, safety, and pleasure and the more disturbing and scary memories, emotions, physical pains, contractions, images, and sensations within the body. In the process of moving between polarities somatically, we encourage a neutralizing effect, much as what happens when we mix hot and cold substances.

Here's an outline for trying the practice yourself:

- Invoke one of the earlier resources and explore it in your body for a few minutes.

- Now choose a challenging memory, emotion, or situation to practice with. Don't start by picking something too major.

- Enter your body and turn toward this challenge, feeling whatever comes up as sensation in your body.

- Titrate out of the experience to a level you can manage to stay present with.

- Next, stay with the emotions, sensations, memories, and images in your body for between fifteen and sixty seconds. Do not stay longer than the set amount of time.

- Now back out of this part of the practice and return to the resource, staying with it until you feel it has been established again. Keep in mind that it's okay for a resource to change and develop as you practice pendulation.

- Pendulate between resourced and contracted places within yourself for two to five rounds, then move to *Savasana* (Corpse Pose) or take a break to integrate the experience.

We can practice pendulation between any set of polarities within ourselves. Pendulating between fear and love is particularly powerful, especially because love acts as such potent medicine for fear. I have witnessed the process of pendulation dissolve or change emotions into something else over time. When explored with love, painful emotions can even become pleasurable, empowering, and at times blissful. And when combined with other forms or resourcing and titration, pendulation allows people to encounter and move through fears, wounds, desires, and aspirations they have been too afraid to encounter before.

Practice 6: Saying Yes to the No

I learned this powerful practice for working with resistance from the late Advaita Vedanta master Arnaud Desjardins, and I have applied it to therapy and yoga practice with potent results. Arnaud taught me that when we encounter a powerful memory, sensation, or emotion, our instinctual response is some degree of contraction in the body. This contraction can be subtle or strong, and it is usually accompanied by some type of corresponding thought. For example: *Things shouldn't be this way* or *I wish things were different*. This is the body's and psyche's instinctual way of saying *no* and protecting themselves against feeling. Even if we consciously wish to explore something or heal ourselves, our unconscious may still be hesitant, afraid, or resistant to open toward it. This *no* arises within us here and there to different degrees, and at times it may serve as a healthy boundary against something that doesn't feel safe or an inner experience that we're not yet ready to explore. At other times, however, the *no* is outdated—it only holds us back from increased freedom.

By learning to say *yes* to this *no*, we compassionately bring space, acceptance, and openness to challenging experiences. In asana, this means feeling into the sensation of *no* as a contraction or resistance in the body and allowing it to be there and soften as we place kind attention on it. We keep saying *yes* with words, our inner attitude, and slight self-adjustments in our posture until we find a small *yes* to our belief that things should be other than they are. This practice shifts our relationship with our contraction, often brings about more space within us, and lessens or changes the contraction itself.

At other times, we cannot say *yes* to the *no* because we feel too frustrated, stuck, resistant, or just not ready to do so. In this case, we try to allow ourselves to say *yes* to *not saying yes to the no*. If we are unable to do that, we can say *yes* to progressive levels of *no* within us. Somatically and psychologically saying *yes* to any amount of internal *no* acts as a kind of emotional asana, and people often report experiencing tremendous relief in being able to let their *no* simply be present in their conscious experience. Finally, just like any other asana, our ability to say *yes* to the *no* grows with gradual and sustained practice over time.

THE YOGA & PSYCHE METHOD:
TEN STEPS FOR APPLYING SOMATIC
TECHNOLOGY TO ASANA PRACTICE

Finally, I want to offer the Yoga & Psyche Method—a synthesis of the applications in this chapter as applied to asana practice. You can use the following steps whether teaching a yoga class, participating in one as a student, practicing at home, or exploring asana as a therapist, client, or dyad partner. These steps are offered as guidelines rather than as a precise sequence. Feel free to modify the instructions to suit the context of the given practice environment:

1. Assume a comfortable seated or standing position. Take a few breaths to relax, and gently scan and bring awareness to the body, noticing any emotion or sensation without trying to change it.

2. Next, invoke an embodied resource—a pleasurable or healing asana, pranayama, nature image, yogic visualization, or a pleasant sensation in the body.

3. Track the sensations of the resource and allow them to move and change. Attend to the sensations while noticing any emotions, images, memories, and insights that arise.

4. Choose an asana to practice with. You might select one you feel resistance to, or one you find more easeful. Both options present distinct benefits. (When repeating this exercise, try both.)

5. Enter the posture and find your edge. Then back out of the pose until you don't experience physical strain but you can still feel the physio-emotional impact of the asana. (Back out of a pose by at least 30 percent, and up to 90 percent or more.)

6. Bring loving attention to the sensations, images, and emotions that arise, titrating 2 to 5 percent deeper into contractions,

resistance, and feelings for short periods of time (between thirty and sixty seconds). Track sensations as they travel through the body.

7. Back out of the asana completely and move into a resourceful, easy, and nurturing pose such as Mountain Pose, Child's Pose (*Balasana*), or seated meditation. Reestablish a sense of resource in the body.

8. Optional step: Reenter, or pendulate, into the asana in step 4, perhaps entering into the emotion or sensation 1 to 5 percent more deeply each time, or choosing to intensify the asana slightly.

9. Again, back out and return to a resourced pose. You can practice pendulation between three and five times, but always end with resourcing (step 2).

10. Finish with *Savasana* (Corpse Pose) or rest.

To summarize, this chapter gives you three key principles, six integrated practices, and a method to consolidate all of them with asana. Everything you find here explores the integration of yoga, psychology, somatics, trauma research, and neuroscience, and you can apply these practices in various contexts: in yoga, therapy, self-inquiry, and dyad practice, whether you are working as a student or teacher. Over time, you will progressively feel the tangible results of these practices and make refinements that suit your own work and personal life.

I offer these tools not as an endpoint but as a foundation for your own discovery. With them, may you explore how somatics, psychology, yoga, trauma studies, and neuroscience work together, support each other, and blend in surprisingly beneficial and potentially evolutionary ways. I encourage you to bring all of your knowledge, uniqueness, and gifts to this developing synthesis.

9

SAVASANA
Integration

Work of the eyes is done, now
Go and do heart-work[1]
RAINER MARIA RILKE, "Turning-Point"

Finally, we arrive at *Savasana*—Corpse Pose—the science and practice of rest and integration. I've synthesized extensive research, useful practices, and my own experience; now it's up to you to integrate it all into your own life. It's time to gather the fruits of your own exploration, insight, healing, and discovery. As I've stated before, yoga gives us incredible maps, and psychology others, but we are the ones who travel the territory.

Personally, I've always felt empowered by this. In yoga, nobody told me what to think, feel, or do; I was merely given instructions to empower my own explorations and experiences. The invitation for us all to do so holds true when it comes to psychological inquiry, and doubly so when we combine the fields of yoga and psychology in our lives. So this is my sincere intention in offering this book: I want to provide you with practical maps, encourage your journey, and celebrate the fruits of our collective inquiry.

YOGA AND PSYCHOLOGY:
1 + 1 = MORE THAN TWO

By integrating these two amazing traditions, we arrive at something greater than either of them alone. Yoga becomes more when it engages psychology, and psychology expands with yoga. And when we add invaluable input from trauma research, somatics, and neuroscience, we weave a union of traditions to create profound potential and possibilities. These include:

- **Integrated Embodiment**   The synthesis of these traditions fosters all levels of embodiment—physical, emotional, and spiritual. When consciousness awakens so thoroughly in the body, we enjoy increased happiness and healing, improved health and well-being, and an enhanced sense of thriving.

- **Yoga Teachers and Students Who Are Informed by Psychology, Somatics, Neuroscience, and Trauma Research** Our practice and teaching begin to naturally include the processing of psychological, somatic, emotional, and traumatic material. When we discover for ourselves how to practice in this way, we bring this capacity to any yoga class or personal activities, and we enjoy additional psychological benefits from our yoga practice.

- **Yogically Informed Approaches to Somatics and Psychology** Drawing upon asana, pranayama, visualization, meditation, and an array of esoteric yoga practices, we expand our understanding of psychology and somatics, extending their scope and effectiveness in our lives. Specifically, we learn to integrate more of our psychological material through the vehicle of yoga.

- **Increased Understanding of the Psychosomatic Dimensions of Yoga**   As students, we often don't know how to work with poses that irritate us or that we want to avoid. We sometimes come to yoga wondering if a given pain is physical, psychological, or both. Integrating yoga and psychology empowers us to discern this for ourselves in the present moment and in the pose, and it enables us to unwind these pains and contractions effectively. Furthermore, we become better able to support others in doing the same for themselves.

- **Psycho-Spiritual Integration**   Classical yoga offers powerful esoteric techniques to enter the body, work with fluctuations of the mind, and explore the spiritual domains of consciousness. Somatics, neuroscience, trauma research, and innovative psychologies offer new tools to effectively explore the various forms of trauma that Western practitioners face. Together, they offer a more complete possibility for us to heal and transform. Their combined methods enable us to safely uncover and explore the images, memories, psychological wounds, and even multigenerational imprints that each of us carry, while simultaneously introducing us to an expanded and more developed spirituality.

CREATING A NEW FIELD TOGETHER

As I've mentioned before, the integration of psychology and yoga does not belong to any of us alone. It belongs to everyone who brings their wisdom, gifts, and heart to this shared journey. And so this book begins and ends with an open invitation to create this new field together, uncovering the endless mysteries of yoga and the deep psyche—not as isolated explorers, but as a community of friends and fellow travelers. I invite you to join us in the dynamic collaboration of our discoveries and developing gifts. Together, we become so much more than any of us will ever become alone.

Patanjali, the compiler of the Yoga Sutras, is often depicted as sitting upon a snake called Ananta. In Sanskrit, this word means "endless," "limitless," "eternal," or "infinite." Just so, yoga and the psyche are without end, and our explorations of them offer perpetual possibility. For this reason, we are always beginners; assuming any type of conclusive mastery or arrival on our journey only prevents our further growth. At the same time, because there is no end point, we are always perfectly situated just as we are, and uniquely gifted to meet the situation in front of us and offer what we have learned to those we are called to care for and support.

I once journeyed through the Himalayas on a quest to discover what enlightenment looks like in the form of female teachers. I had the tremendous fortune to visit with the late Vimala Thakar, an Advaita master in the lineage of Jiddu Krishnamurti. When I asked this exemplary elder how she had met the challenges on her lifelong path of yoga and deep inquiry, she responded:

> My love of life and the urge to discover the truth firsthand
> sustained me. I had read so much, but I could not be satisfied
> in borrowing anyone's version of truth. I would probe and
> probe until the light dawned on me. Living here in India—
> a woman unmarried—it was not a path of roses. There
> were many difficulties and handicaps. But a revolutionary
> cannot have the luxury of defeat: pessimism, negativity.
> Never. Difficulties can be converted into opportunities,
> challenges into the call for more creativity. Everything in life
> has two aspects: if you know how to use it, it becomes an
> advantage, and if you don't know how to use it, it becomes
> a disadvantage. That's what I have done, my dear. For every
> challenge I received, I would say, "This is a love letter from
> the Divine, and I must find an answer from within."[2]

I see the call to integrate yoga and psychology as a love letter, too. I hope you receive this invitation freely and choose to explore what happens when you bring your full self to this shared inquiry. As we each receive this love letter and share with each other the responses we discover with each other, we connect in a new and abundant field of our own creation. With folded hands and outstretched arms, I share this book as an offering into this new field, dream, and vision.

ACKNOWLEDGMENTS

I want to acknowledge my deep gratitude to my spiritual teacher, Lee Lozowick, and his guru, Yogi Ramsuratkumar. Both of these masters were powerful transmitters of tantric yoga whose kindness and wisdom continue to inspire me today. I also want to thank Arnaud Desjardins, the late Advaita Vedanta master, and the Sufi master Llewellyn Vaughan-Lee, whose teachings and presence have impacted me profoundly.

My hatha yoga training was most strongly influenced by Bhavani Maki, who is the founder of Yoga Hanalei in Kaua'i. Many other yoga teachers in the field who have become cherished friends and colleagues have deeply influenced me and taught me through our exchange, including Nubia Teixeira, Janice Gates, Sally Kempton, and Anne Cushman.

As a graduate student at the California Institute of Integral Studies (and later as a professor), I encountered a number of psychological visionaries who helped me along the way. Peter Levine's Somatic Experiencing training (which I completed in 2006) has proven invaluable—I've used it extensively in my Yoga & Psyche trainings, my private psychotherapy practice, my personal practice, and now this book.

Through the International Yoga & Psyche Conference in 2014, I met a number of important influences in my life. I have been deeply touched by Angela Farmer, Rama Jyoti Vernon, Eleanor Criswell, and Yogi Amrit Desai, among others. I have also learned a great deal from my clients, graduate students, the participants in my programs, and those who have entrusted me to their care at different levels as I continue to develop this body of work. I also want to acknowledge a neuroscientist, yoga teacher, and "rock-star" friend, Gabriel Axel, with whom I subsequently coedited the volume *Proceedings of the Yoga & Psyche Conference (2014)*. Gabriel also coauthored the "Yoga, Science, and the Brain" chapter in this book, and his knowledge adds a crucial dimension to this inquiry.

Various teachers of diverse paths have blessed and supported me over the years. These include the late Georg Feuerstein, John Welwood, Claudio Naranjo, and A. H. Almaas (Hameed Ali). I also want to thank Holly Adler, Kim Burris, Dhyana Justl, Raia Kogan, Adriana Portillo, Haley Roth, Lynsie Seely, Kristine Tom, and Lauren Weiss for their friendship and assistance with the research presented here. Additionally, this work would not be possible without Jorge Ferrer, Hannah Gottsegen, Suraya Keating, Anastasi Mavrides, Karen Motan, Simone Thurston, Vipassana Esbjorn-Hargens, Marianne Costa, and so many other wise, dear, and brilliant friends.

Tami Simon found me years ago when I was living on my teacher's ashram and asked me to write books for Sounds True. The whole crew has supported me impeccably through my publishing journey. My editors are brilliant, and the company is an expression of deep spiritual integrity.

My father, Herb Caplan, brought me into the world and has showered me with his pride and generosity throughout the years. When I was a young child, my mother (Mollie Caplan, who died a number of years ago) wrote in her diary that I would one day become an author, and I want to thank her for planting that seed in me.

I invoke the blessings of each of these individuals as I birth this book into the world, and I thank each of them for their unique gift and contribution to my life. May I accurately represent their teachings and transmissions in my own work integrating the fields of yoga and psychology.

NOTES

Introduction

1. Emily Dickinson, "Not knowing when the dawn will come," in *The Complete Poems of Emily Dickinson* (Boston: Little, Brown, 1924), bartleby. com/113.

2. In this book I speak of the *Western* psyche simply because I am most experienced and competent in addressing people in the West. Having said that, I strongly support people from around the world taking insights and practices from this book and applying and integrating them into their own religious, spiritual, and cultural contexts.

Chapter 1: The Marriage of Ancient Wisdom and Depth Psychology

1. The number of years that psychology has existed varies widely from source to source.

2. Mircea Eliade, *Patanjali and Yoga*, trans. Charles Lam Markmann (New York: Schocken Books, 1975).

3. Georg Feuerstein, *The Yoga Tradition: Its History, Literature, Philosophy, and Practice* (Prescott, AZ: Hohm Press, 1998), 62.

4. Edwin Bryant, *The Yoga Sutras of Patanjali* (New York: North Point Press, 2009).

5. "2016 Yoga in America Study Conducted by *Yoga Journal* and Yoga Alliance," Yoga Alliance, January 13, 2016, yogaalliance. org/2016yogainamericastudy.

6. Ibid.

7. Online Etymology Dictionary, s.v. "psyche," by Douglas Harper, etymonline.com/index.php?term=psyche.

8. Carl Gustav Jung, *Psychology and Religion: East and West*, trans. R.F.C. Hull (Princeton, NJ: Yale University Press, 1938), 500.

9. Carl Gustav Jung, *Civilization in Transition: The Collected Works of C.G. Jung, Volume 10*, eds. Michael Fordham and Gerhard Adler, trans. R.F.C. Hull (New York: Routledge, 1964), 4450.

10. Carl Gustav Jung, *Modern Man in Search of a Soul* trans. Carl F. Baynes (New York: Routledge Classics, 2001), 35.

11. Mariana Caplan, Adriana Portillo, and Lynsie Seely, "Yoga Psychotherapy: The Integration of Western Psychological Theory and Ancient Yogic Wisdom," *Journal of Transpersonal Psychology* 45, no. 2 (2013), 139–158.

12. "Yoga for Anxiety and Depression," Harvard Mental Health Letter published April 2009, updated September 18, 2017, health.harvard.edu/ mind-and-mood/yoga-for-anxiety-and-depression.

13. Caplan et al., "Yoga Psychotherapy," 139–158.

14. Lourdes P. Dale et al., "Yoga Workshop Impacts Psychological Functioning and Mood of Women with Self-Reported History of Eating Disorders," *Eating Disorders: The Journal of Treatment & Prevention* 17, no. 5 (2009): 422–434, doi: 10.1080/10640260903210222.

15. Caplan et al., "Yoga Psychotherapy," 139–158.

16. P.A. Kinser et al., "Feasibility, Acceptability, and Effects of Gentle Hatha Yoga for Women with Major Depression: Findings from a Randomized Controlled Mixed-Methods Study," *Archives of Psychiatric Nursing* 27, no. 3 (2013): 137–147, doi: 10.1016/j.apnu.2013.01.003.

17. Bo Forbes et al., "Using Integrative Yoga Therapeutics in the Treatment of Comorbid Anxiety and Depression," *International Journal of Yoga Therapy* 18, no. 1 (2008): 87–95, EBSCOhost.

18. Richard C. Miller, "The Breath of Life: Through the Practice of Pranayama, the Regulation of the Breath, We Can Learn to Bring Forth and Direct the Spiritual Energy That Underlies All Life," *Yoga Journal* 116 (May/June 1994): 82, EBSCOhost.

19. Lloyd Lalande et al., "Breathwork: An Additional Treatment Option for Depression and Anxiety?" *Journal of Contemporary Psychotherapy* 42, no. 2 (2012): 113–119.

20. David Shapiro and Karen Cline, "Mood Changes Associated with Iyengar Yoga Practices: A Pilot Study," *International Journal of Yoga Therapy* 14, no. 1 (2004): 35–44, EBSCOhost.

21. Chris C. Streeter et al., "Effects of Yoga Versus Walking on Mood, Anxiety, and Brain GABA Levels: A Randomized Controlled MRS Study," *Journal of Alternative and Complementary Medicine* 16, no. 11 (2010): 1145–1152, doi: 10.1089/acm.2010.0007.

22. E. A. Impett et al., "Minding the Body: Yoga, Embodiment, and Well-Being," *Sexuality Research and Social Policy* 3, no. 4 (2006): 39–48, doi: 10.1525/srsp.2006.3.4.39.

23. Amy Swart, "Partner Yoga for Establishing Boundaries in Relationship: A Transpersonal Somatic Approach," *International Journal of Yoga Therapy* 21 (2011): 123–128, EBSCOhost.

24. Sarah W. Lazar et al., "Functional Brain Mapping of the Relaxation Response and Meditation," *NeuroReport* 11, no. 7 (May 15, 2000): 1581–1585, massgeneral.org/bhi/assets/pdfs/publications/lazar_2000_neuroreport.pdf.

25. Danielle V. Shelov et al., "A Pilot Study Measuring the Impact of Yoga on the Trait of Mindfulness," *Behavioral and Cognitive Psychotherapy* 37, no. 5 (2009): 595–598, doi: 10.1017/S1352465809990361.

26. Mark Epstein, "Meditative Transformations of Narcissism," *Journal of Transpersonal Psychology* 18, no, 2 (1986): 143–158, atpweb.org/jtparchive/trps-18-86-02-143.pdf.

27. Britta K. Hölzel et al., "How Does Mindfulness Meditation Work? Proposing Mechanisms of Action from a Conceptual and Neural Perspective." *Perspectives on Psychological Science* 6, no. 6 (2011): 537–559, doi: 10.1177/1745691611419671.

28. For an in-depth look at yoga's evolution and migration, see Georg Feuerstein's *The Yoga Tradition: Its History, Literature, Philosophy, and Practice* (Prescott, AZ: Hohm Press, 1998) and Philip Goldberg's *American Veda: From Emerson and the Beatles to Yoga and Meditation—How Indian Spirituality Changed the West* (New York: Harmony Books, 2010).

29. Jung's quote is from Roger Walsh's "The Search for Synthesis," *Journal of Humanistic Psychology* 32, no.1 (1992): 19–45.

30. Stephen Cope, *Yoga and the Quest for the True Self* (New York: Bantam, 2000), xv.

Chapter 2: Why Yoga Needs Psychology

1. Stephen Cope, *Yoga and the Quest for the True Self* (New York: Bantam, 2000), xiii.

2. Carl Gustav Jung, "The Philosophical Tree," trans. and ed. Gerhard Adler, in *The Collected Works of C.G. Jung, Vol. 13, Alchemical Studies* (New York: Routledge, 1945), 335.

3. John Welwood called these "relational wounds" in private dialogues with me during March of 2010. These ideas are further discussed in: *Perfect Love, Imperfect Relationships: Healing the Wound of the Heart* (Boston: Trumpeter, 2006).

Chapter 3: Why Psychology Needs Yoga

1. Rama Jyoti Vernon. Keynote address at the International Yoga & Psyche Conference, San Francisco, CA, February, 18, 2014.

2. Marc Halpern, "Ayurvedic Yoga Therapy: An Overview with Case Study," *International Journal of Yoga Therapy* 18 (2008): 25–30.

3. Roger Walsh et al., "Medicate or Meditate?" *Lion's Roar*, March 1, 2009, lionsroar.com/medicate-or-meditate-2.

Chapter 4: Psychology: A New Western Spirituality

1. Carl Gustav Jung, *C.G. Jung Letters, Volume 1: 1906–1950*, eds. Gerhard Adler and Aniela Jaffé, trans. R.F.C. Hull (Princeton, NJ: Princeton University Press, 1973), 33.

2. Mariana Caplan and Gabriel Axel, *Proceedings of the Yoga & Psyche Conference (2014)* (Newcastle upon Tyne, England: Cambridge Scholars Publishing, 2015).

3. Mariana Caplan, Glenn Hartelius, and Mary Ann Rardin, "Contemporary Viewpoints on Transpersonal Psychology," *Journal of Transpersonal Psychology* 35, no. 2 (2003): 143–162.

   See also: Glenn Hartelius, Mariana Caplan, and Mary Ann Rardin, "Transpersonal Psychology: Defining the Past, Divining the Future," *Humanistic Psychologist* 35, no. 2 (2007): 135–160.

4. A summary of the AQAL model and other works of Ken Wilber can be found at kenwilber.com/writings/read_pdf/34.

5. Ibid.

6. Ibid.

7. I heard Joanna Macy give this public talk at the Jennifer Berezan "Song for All Beings" concert on February 26, 2017, in San Rafael, California.

8. From notes I jotted down during a talk Ram Dass gave at Open Secret Bookstore in San Rafael, California, circa 1998.

9. Sutra 2:12 is from: B.K.S. Iyengar, *Light on the Yoga Sutras of Patanjali* (London and San Francisco: Thorsons, 1996).

Chapter 5: Yoga, Science, and the Brain

1. Timothy Rasinski and Lorraine Griffith, *Building Fluency through Practice and Performance* (Huntington Beach, CA: Shell Education, 2008), 64.

2. Sara W. Lazar et al., "Meditation Experience Is Associated with Increased Cortical Thickness," *NeuroReport* 16, no. 17 (2005): 1893–1897, doi: 10.1097/01.wnr.0000186598.66243.19.

   See also: Britta K. Hölzel et al., "Mindfulness Practice Leads to Increases in Regional Brain Grey-Matter Density," *Psychiatry Research* 191, no. 1 (2011): 36–43, doi: 10.1016/j.pscychresns.2010.08.006.

   See also: Rinkske A. Gotink et al., "Mindfulness and Mood Stimulate Each Other in an Upward Spiral: a Mindful Walking Intervention Using Experience Sampling," *Mindfulness* 7, no. 5 (2016), doi: 10.1007/s12671-016-0550-8.

3. Mehmet Somel et al., "Transcriptional Neoteny in the Human Brain," *Proceedings of the National Academy of Sciences* 106, no. 14 (2009): 5743–5748, doi: 10.1073/pnas.0900544106.

4. Mihovil Pletikos et al., "Temporal Specification and Bilaterality of Human Neocortical Topographic Gene Expression," *Neuron* 81, no. 2 (2014): 321–332, doi: 10.1016/j.neuron.2013.11.018.

5. Georg Northoff et al., "Self-Referential Processing in Our Brain—A Meta-Analysis of Imaging Studies on the Self," *NeuroImage* 31, no. 1 (2006): 440–457, doi: 10.1016/j.neuroimage.2005.12.002.

   See also: Pengmin Qin and Georg Northoff, "How is Our Self Related to Midline Regions and the Default-Mode Network?" *NeuroImage* 57, no. 3 (2011): 1221–33, doi: 10.1016/j.neuroimage.2011.05.028.

6. Yi-Yuan Tang, Britta Hölzel, and Michael Posner, "The Neuroscience of Mindfulness Meditation," *Nature Reviews Neuroscience* 16, no. 4 (2015): 213–225, doi: 10.1038/nrn3916.

   See also: Xiyao Xie et al., "How Do You Make Me Feel Better? Social Cognitive Emotion Regulation and the Default Mode Network," *NeuroImage* 134 (2016): 270–280, doi: 10.1016/j.neuroimage.2016.04.015.

7. Stephen W. Porges, "The Polyvagal Theory: New Insights into Adaptive Reactions of the Autonomic Nervous System," *Cleveland Clinic Journal of Medicine* 76, Supplement 2 (2009): S86–S90, doi: 10.3949/ccjm.76.s2.17.

8. Blaine Ditto, Marie Eclache, and Natalie Goldman, "Short-Term Autonomic and Cardiovascular Effects of Mindfulness Body-Scan Meditation," *Annals of Behavioral Medicine* 32, no. 3 (2006): 227–234, doi: 10.1207/s15324796abm3203_9.

See also: C. K. Peng et al., "Heart Rate Dynamics During Three Forms of Meditation," *International Journal of Cardiology* 95, no.1 (2004): 19–27, doi: 10.1016/j.ijcard.2003.02.006.

9. Peter Vestergaard-Poulsen et al., "Long-Term Meditation Is Associated with Increased Gray-Matter Density in the Brain Stem," *NeuroReport* 20, no. 2 (2009): 170–174, doi: 10.1097/WNR.0b013e328320012a.

10. Christopher M. Masi et al., "Respiratory Sinus Arrhythmia and Diseases of Aging: Obesity, Diabetes Mellitus, and Hypertension," *Biological Psychology* 74, no. 2 (2007): 212–223.

11. Junichiro Hayano et al., "Respiratory Sinus Arrhythmia: A Phenomenon Improving Pulmonary Gas Exchange and Circulatory Efficiency," *Circulation* 94, no. 4 (1996): 842–847, doi: 10.1161/01.cir.94.4.842.

12. Lisa M. Diamond et al., "Attachment Style, Vagal Tone, and Empathy During Mother-Adolescent Interactions," *Journal of Research on Adolescence* 22, no. 1 (2012): 165–184, doi: 10.1111/j.1532-7795.2011.00762.x.

13. Julian Koenig et al., "Resting State Vagal Tone in Borderline Personality Disorder: A Meta-Analysis," *Progress in Neuro-Psychopharmacology and Biological Psychiatry* 64 (2016): 18–26, doi: 10.1016/j.pnpbp.2015.07.002.

14. Bethany E. Kok et al., "How Positive Emotions Build Physical Health: Perceived Positive Social Connections Account for the Upward Spiral Between Positive Emotions and Vagal Tone," *Psychological Science* 24, no. 7 (2013): 1123–1132, doi: 10.1177/0956797612470827.

15. Elisa Raffaella Ferrè et al., "Anchoring the Self to the Body: Vestibular Contribution to the Sense of Self," *Psychological Science* 25, no. 11 (2014): 2106–2108, doi: 10.1177/0956797614547917.

16. Tang, Hölzel, and Posner, "The Neuroscience of Mindfulness Meditation," 213–225

See also: Tim Gard et al., "Potential Self-Regulatory Mechanisms of Yoga for Psychological Health," *Frontiers in Human Neuroscience* 8 (2014): 770, doi: 10.3389/fnhum.2014.00770.

17. Hölzel et al. "Mindfulness Practice Leads to Increases in Regional Brain Grey-Matter Density," 36–43.

18. Kevin N. Ochsner and James J. Gross, "The Cognitive Control of Emotion," *Trends in Cognitive Sciences* 9, no. 5 (2005): 242–249, doi: 10.1016/j.tics.2005.03.010.

19. Britta K. Hölzel, "Stress Reduction Correlates with Structural Changes in the Amygdala," *Social Cognitive and Affective Neuroscience* 5, no. 1 (2010): 11–17, doi: 10.1093/scan/nsp034.

20. Olaf Blanke, "Multisensory Brain Mechanisms of Bodily Self-Consciousness," *Nature Reviews Neuroscience* 13, no. 8 (2012): 556–571, doi: 10.1038/nrn3292.

    See also: Michael. S. Graziano and Taylor W. Webb, "The Attention Schema Theory: A Mechanistic Account of Subjective Awareness," *Frontiers in Psychology* 6 (2015): 500, doi: 10.3389/fpsyg.2015.00500.

21. Wendy Hasenkamp et al., "Mind Wandering and Attention During Focused Meditation: A Fine-Grained Temporal Analysis of Fluctuating Cognitive States," *NeuroImage* 59, no. 1 (2012): 750–760, doi: 10.1016/j.neuroimage.2011.07.008.

    See also: Wendy Hasenkamp and Lawrence W. Barsalou, "Effects of Meditation Experience on Functional Connectivity of Distributed Brain Networks," *Frontiers in Human Neuroscience* 6 (2012): 38, doi: 10.3389/fnhum.2012.00038.

22. Tang, Hölzel, and Posner, "The Neuroscience of Mindfulness Meditation," 213–225

23. Judson A. Brewer et al., "Meditation Experience Is Associated with Differences in Default Mode Network Activity and Connectivity," *Proceedings of the National Academy of Sciences of the United States of America* 108, no. 50 (2011): 20254–20259, doi: 10.1073/pnas.1112029108.

    See also: Marco Sperduti et al., "A Neurocognitive Model of Meditation Based on Activation Likelihood Estimation (ALE) Meta-Analysis," *Consciousness and Cognition* 21 (2012): 269–276, doi: 10.1016/j.concog.2011.09.019.

24. Hasenkamp and Barsalou, "Effects of Meditation Experience on Functional Connectivity of Distributed Brain Networks," 38.

25. Sperduti et al., "A Neurocognitive Model of Meditation Based on Activation Likelihood Estimation (ALE) Meta-Analysis," 269–276.

26. Tang, Hölzel, and Posner, "The Neuroscience of Mindfulness Meditation," 213–225

    See also: Gard et al., "Potential Self-Regulatory Mechanisms of Yoga for Psychological Health," 770.

27. Norman A.S. Farb et al., "Attending to the Present: Mindfulness Meditation Reveals Distinct Neural Modes of Self-Reference," *Social Cognitive and Affective Neuroscience* 2, no. 4 (2007): 313–322, doi: 10.1093/scan/nsm030.

    See also: Brewer et al., "Meditation Experience Is Associated with Differences in Default Mode Network Activity and Connectivity," 20254–20259.

28. Antonio R. Damasio et al., "The Somatic Marker Hypothesis and the Possible Functions of the Prefrontal Cortex [and Discussion]," *Philosophical Transactions of the Royal Society of London B: Biological Sciences* 351, no. 1346 (1996): 1413–1420, doi: 10.1098/rstb.1996.0125.

29. Kevin N. Ochsner et al., "For Better or for Worse: Neural Systems Supporting the Cognitive Down-and-Up-Regulation of Negative Emotion," *NeuroImage* 23, no. 2 (2004): 483–499, doi: 10.1016/j.neuroimage.2004.06.030.

30. Xie et al., "How Do You Make Me Feel Better? Social Cognitive Emotion Regulation and the Default Mode Network," 270–280.

31. Brewer, et al., "Meditation Experience Is Associated with Differences in Default Mode Network Activity and Connectivity," 20254–20259.

32. Hasenkamp and Barsalou, "Effects of Meditation Experience on Functional Connectivity of Distributed Brain Networks," 38.

33. Hölzel et al., "How Does Mindfulness Meditation Work? Proposing Mechanisms of Action from a Conceptual and Neural Perspective," 537–559.

34. Tang, Hölzel, and Posner, "The Neuroscience of Mindfulness Meditation," 213–225

35. Paul Rozin and Edward B. Royzman, "Negativity Bias, Negativity Dominance, and Contagion," *Personality and Social Psychology Review* 5, no. 4, (2001): 296–320, doi: 10.1207/s15327957pspr0504_2.

    See also: G. Elliott Wimmer and Daphna Shohamy, "Preference by Association: How Memory Mechanisms in the Hippocampus Bias Decisions," *Science* 338, no. 6104 (2012): 270–273, doi: 10.1126/science.1223252.

Chapter 6: How Somatic Psychology Changes the Game

1. Carl Gustav Jung, "Psychological Factors Determining Human Behavior," *Factors Determining Human Behavior* (Boston: Harvard Tercentenary Publications, 1937).

2. Thomas Hanna, *Bodies in Revolt: A Primer in Somatic Thinking* (New York, NY: Holt, Rinehart, Winston, 1970), 35.

3. Thomas Hanna, "What Is Somatics?" in *Bone, Breath, and Gesture: Practices of Embodiment, Volume 1*, ed. Don Hanlon Johnson (Berkeley, CA: North Atlantic Books, 1995), 343.

4. Bill Bowen, *Somatic Resourcing* (Portland, OR: PPT Publishing, 2009), 6.

5. Laura Steckler and Courtenay Young, "Depression and Body Psychotherapy," *International Journal of Psychotherapy* 13, no. 2 (2009): 32–41, courtenay-young.co.uk/courtenay/articles/Steckler_Young_Depression_BP.pdf.

6. Margit Koemeda-Lutz et al., "Evaluation of the Effectiveness of Body Psychotherapy in Outpatient Settings (EEBP): A Multicenter Study in Germany and Switzerland," *Psychother. Psych. Med. Psychosom.* 206, no. 56 (2006): 480–487, hakomiinstitute.com/Forum/Issue19-21/12EABPresearch.art2.pdf.

7. Giovanni Lopez, "Why Verbal Psychotherapy Is Not Enough to Treat Post-Traumatic Stress Disorder: A Biosystemic Approach to Stress Debriefing," *Body, Movement, and Dance in Psychotherapy* 6, no. 2 (2011): 129–143, doi: 10.1080/17432979.2011.583060.

8. Cynthia Price, "Body-Oriented Therapy in Recovery from Child Sexual Abuse: An Efficacy Study," *Alternative Therapies in Health and Medicine* 11, no. 5 (2005): 46–57.

   See also: Cynthia J. Price, et al., "Mindful Awareness in Body-Oriented Therapy for Female Veterans with Post-Traumatic Stress Disorder Taking Prescription Analgesics for Chronic Pain: A Feasibility Study," *Alternative Therapies in Health and Medicine* 13, no. 6 (2007): 32–40.

9. Anodea Judith, *Eastern Body, Western Mind: Psychology and the Chakra System as a Path to the Self* (Berkeley, CA: Celestial Arts, 2004), 14–15, 54.

10. Peter Levine, *In an Unspoken Voice: How the Body Releases Trauma and Restores Goodness* (Berkeley, CA: North Atlantic Books, 2012), 278.

11. Mother Teresa, *Mother Teresa Come Be My Light*, ed. Brian Kolodiejchuk (New York: Crown Publishing Group, 2009), 230.

12. Nikos Kazantzakis, *Report to Greco*, trans. Peter A. Bien (New York: Simon & Schuster, 1965), 45.

13. From Chögyam Trungpa's unpublished writings. This quote was adapted from a talk given by John Welwood at the California Institute of Integral Studies in San Francisco in 2001.

Chapter 7: Overcoming Trauma with Somatics and Yoga

1. Bessel van der Kolk, *The Body Keeps the Score* (New York: Viking Penguin Books, 2014), 238.

2. Robert Scaer, *The Body Bears the Burden: Trauma, Dissociation, and Disease, Second Edition* (New York: Routledge, 2007), 109.

3. Ibid., 153.

4. Bessel van der Kolk, "Developmental Trauma Disorder: Towards a Rational Diagnosis for Children with Complex Trauma Histories," *Psychiatric Annals* 35, no. 5 (May 2005): 401. van der Kolk is also referencing the research of Alexandra Cook and Joseph Spinazolla et al.: "Complex Trauma in Children and Adolescents," *Psychiatric Annals* 35, no. 5 (May 2005).

5. Babette Rothschild, *The Body Remembers: The Psychophysiology of Trauma and Trauma Treatment* (New York: W.W. Norton & Company, 2000), 6.

6. Peter Levine, *In an Unspoken Voice*, 131.

7. Bessel van der Kolk et al., "The Assessment and Treatment of Complex PTSD," *Traumatic Stress,* ed. Rachel Yehuda (Arlington, VA: American Psychiatric Press, 2001), 11.

8. van der Kolk, *he Body Keeps the Score*, 203.

9. Here I'm restating some of the research noted in chapter 1, as well as: Caplan et al., "Yoga Psychotherapy," 139–158.

10. Sita Martin, T*he Hunger of Love: Versions of the Ramayana* (Kanyakumari, India: Yogi Ramsuratkumar Manthralayam Trust, 1995).

11. Rick Hanson, *Buddha's Brain: The Practical Neuroscience of Happiness, Love, and Wisdom* (Oakland, CA: New Harbinger Publications, 2009), 14.

12. Peter Levine, *In an Unspoken Voice*, 37.

Chapter 8: The Yoga & Psyche Method Toolbox

1. Lee Lozowick's words are from a personal meeting in 1995 at the Hohm Community Ashram when it was in Prescott, Arizona.

2. The list of "feeling" words is from the 2008 training manual for the Somatic Experiencing and Trauma Institute's certification program.

3. Hanna, "What Is Somatics?" 343.

Chapter 9: Savasana: Integration

1. Rainer Maria Rilke, "Turning-Point," *The Selected Poetry of Rainer Maria Rilke*, trans. and ed. Stephen Mitchell (New York: Vintage Books, 1989), 134–135.

2. Vimala Thakar's words of wisdom are from a personal interview at her residence in Dalhousie, India, in June 2001.

REFERENCES

BOOKS

American Psychiatric Association, ed. *Diagnostic and Statistical Manual of Mental Disorders, Fifth Edition*. Washington, DC: American Psychiatric Association Publishing, 2013.

Amthor, Frank. *Neuroscience for Dummies*. Hoboken, NJ: John Wiley & Sons, 2012.

Bainbridge Cohen, Bonnie. *Sensing, Feeling, and Action: The Experiential Anatomy of Body-Mind Centering, Third Edition*. Northampton, MA: Contact Edition, 2012.

Boon, Suzette, Kathy Steele, and Onno Van Der Hart. *Coping with Trauma-Related Dissociation: Skills Training for Patients and Their Therapists*. New York: W.W. Norton, 2011.

Bowen, Bill. *Somatic Resourcing: Psychotherapy Through the Body*. Portland, OR: PPT, 2009. Ebook.

Bryant, Edwin. *The Yoga Sūtras of Patañjali*. New York, NY: North Point Press, 2009.

Caplan, Mariana. *Eyes Wide Open: Cultivating Discernment on the Spiritual Path*. Boulder, CO: Sounds True, 2009.

_____. *Halfway Up the Mountain: The Error of Premature Claims to Enlightenment*. Chino Valley, AZ: Hohm Press, 1999.

_____. *The Guru Question: The Perils and Rewards of Choosing a Spiritual Teacher*. Boulder, CO: Sounds True, 2010.

_____. *To Touch Is to Live: The Need for Genuine Affection in an Increasingly Impersonal World*. Prescott, AZ: Hohm Press, 2002.

_____. *When Sons and Daughters Choose Alternative Lifestyles*. Prescott, AZ: Hohm Press, 1997.

Caplan, Mariana, and Gabriel Axel, eds. *Proceedings of the Yoga & Psyche Conference (2014)*. Cambridge, UK: Cambridge Scholars, 2015.

Cope, Stephen. *Yoga and the Quest for the True Self*. New York: Bantam, 1999.

Cope, Stephen, ed. *Will Yoga & Meditation Really Change My Life?: Personal Stories from America's Leading Teachers*. North Adams, MA: Storey, 2003.

Corrigall, Jenny, Helen Payne, and Heward Wilkinson, eds. *About a Body: Working with the Embodied Mind in Psychotherapy*. London: Routledge, 2006.

Coward, Harold. *Yoga and Psychology: Language, Memory, and Mysticism*. Albany, NY: State University of New York Press, 2002.

Damasio, Antonio. *The Feeling of What Happens: Body and Emotion in the Making of Consciousness*. New York: Harcourt Brace, 1999.

————. *Looking for Spinoza: Joy, Sorrow, and the Feeling Brain*. Orlando, FL: Harcourt, 2003.

Desikachar, T.K.V. The Heart of Yoga: Developing a Personal Practice. Rochester, VT: Inner Traditions International, 1995.

Desjardins, Arnaud. *The Jump into Life*. Translated by Kathleen Kennedy. Prescott, AZ: Hohm Press, 1994.

————. *Toward the Fullness of Life*. Translated by Kathleen Kennedy. Chino Valley, AZ: Hohm Press, 2015.

Eliade, Mircea. *Yoga: Immortality and Freedom.* Translated by Willard R. Trask. Princeton, NJ: Princeton University Press, 1970.

————. *Patanjali and Yoga*. Translated by Charles Lam Markmann. New York: Schocken Books, 1975.

Emerson, David. *Yoga & Mindfulness Therapy Workbook for Clinicians and Clients*. Eau Claire, WI: PESI Publishing and Media, 2014.

Emerson, David, and Elizabeth Hopper. *Overcoming Trauma through Yoga: Reclaiming Your Body*. Berkeley, CA: North Atlantic, 2011.

Feuerstein, Georg. *Tantra: The Path of Ecstasy*. Boston: Shambhala, 1998.

————. *The Deeper Dimension of Yoga*. Boston: Shambhala, 2003.

————. *The Philosophy of Classical Yoga*. Rochester, VT: Inner Traditions International, 1996.

————. *The Yoga Tradition: Its History, Literature, Philosophy, and Practice*. Prescott, AZ: Hohm Press, 1998.

Forbes, Bo. *Yoga for Emotional Balance: Simple Practices to Help Relieve Anxiety and Depression*. Boston: Shambhala, 2011.

Gerbarg, Patricia L., and Richard P. Brown. "Mind-Body Practices for Recovery from Sexual Trauma," *Surviving Sexual Violence: A Guide to Recovery and Empowerment*, Thema Bryant-Davis, ed. 199–216. Lanham, MD: Rowman & Littlefield, 2011.

Goldberg, Philip. *American Veda: From Emerson and the Beatles to Yoga and Meditation—How Indian Spirituality Changed the West*. New York: Harmony Books, 2010.

Ghose, Aurobindo. *Integral Yoga: Sri Aurobindo's Teaching and Method of Practice* . Twin Lakes, WI: Lotus Press, 1998.

Grof, Stanislav, and Christina Grof. *Holotropic Breathwork: A New Approach to Self-Exploration and Therapy*. Albany, NY: State University of New York Press, 2010.

Hanna, Thomas *Bodies in Revolt: A Primer in Somatic Thinking*. New York: Holt, Rinehart and Winston, 1970.

————. *Somatics: Reawakening the Mind's Control of Movement, Flexibility, and Health*. Boston: Da Capo Press, 1988.

Hanson, Rick, and Richard Mendius. *Buddha's Brain: The Practical Neuroscience of Happiness, Love, and Wisdom*. Oakland, CA: New Harbinger Publications, 2009.

Hartley, Linda. *Somatic Psychology: Body, Mind, and Meaning*. Philadelphia: Whurr Publishers Ltd., 2004.

Heller, Laurence, and Aline LaPierre. *Healing Developmental Trauma: How Early Trauma Affects Self-Regulation, Self-Image, and the Capacity for Relationship*. Berkeley, CA: North Atlantic Books, 2012.

Iyengar, B.K.S. *Light on the Yoga Sutras of Patanjali*. New Delhi, India: HarperCollins India, 2005.

————. *Light on Yoga*. New York: Schocken Books, 1979.

Johnson, Don Hanlon, ed. *Bone, Breath, and Gesture: Practices of Embodiment, Volume 1*. Berkeley, CA: North Atlantic Books, 1995.

Judith, Anodea. *Eastern Body, Western Mind: Psychology and the Chakra System as a Path to the Self, Revised Edition</ital.>*. Berkeley, CA: Celestial Arts, 2004.

Jung, Carl Gustav. *Civilization in Transition: The Collected Works of C.G. Jung, Volume 10*, eds. Michael Fordham and Gerhard Adler, translated by R.F.C. Hull New York: Routledge, 1964.

————. *Modern Man in Search of a Soul*. Translated by William Stanley Dell. London: K. Paul, Trench, Trubner, 1933.

————. *Psychology and Religion: East and West*. Ed. Gerhard Adler and translated by R.F.C. Hull. Princeton, NJ: Yale University Press, 1938.

————. *The Psychology of Kundalini Yoga: Notes of the Seminar Given in 1932 by C. G. Jung*. Ed. by Sonu Shamdasani. Princeton, NJ: Princeton University Press, 1996.

Kalsched, Donald. *The Inner World of Trauma: Archetypal Defenses of the Personal Spirit*. London: Routledge, 1996.

Kazantzakis, Nikos. *Report to Greco*. Translated by Peter Bien. New York: Simon & Schuster, 1965.

Kempton, Sally. *Awakening Shakti: The Transformative Power of the Goddesses of Yoga*. Boulder, CO: Sounds True, 2013.

————. *Meditation for the Love of It: Enjoying Your Own Deepest Experience*. Boulder, CO: Sounds True, 2011.

Kinsley, David. *Tantric Visions of the Divine Feminine*. Berkeley, CA: University of California Press, 1997.

Kurtz, Ron. *Body-Centered Psychotherapy: The Hakomi Method*. Mendocino, CA: LifeRhythm Publication, 2007.

Levine, Peter A. *In an Unspoken Voice: How the Body Releases Trauma and Restores Goodness*. Berkeley, CA: North Atlantic Books, 2010.

————. *Healing Trauma: A Pioneering Program for Restoring the Wisdom of Your Body*. Boulder, CO: Sounds True, 2008.

————. *Trauma and Memory: Brain and Body in a Search for the Living Past: A Practical Guide for Understanding and Working with Traumatic Memory*. Berkeley, CA: North Atlantic Books, 2015.

————. *Waking the Tiger: Healing Trauma*. Berkeley, Calif.: North Atlantic Books, 1997.

Lowen, Alexander. *Bioenergetics: The Revolutionary Therapy that Uses the Language of the Body to Heal the Problems of the Mind.* New York: Penguin, 1994.

Lozowick, Lee. *Feast or Famine: Teachings on Mind and Emotions.* Chino Valley, AZ: Hohm Press, 2008.

_____. *The Alchemy of Transformation.* Chino Valley, AZ: Hohm Press, 1996.

Macnaughton, Ian, ed. *Body, Breath & Consciousness: A Somatics Anthology.* Berkeley, CA: North Atlantic Books, 2004.

Maki, Bhavani Silvia. *The Yogi's Roadmap: Patanjali Yoga Sutra as a Journey to Self Realization.* Hanalei, HI: Viveka Press, 2013.

Martin, Sita. *The Hunger of Love: Versions of the Ramayana.* Kanyakumari, India: Yogi Ramsuratkumar Manthralayam Trust, 1995.

Merton, Robert K. ed. *Factors Determining Human Behavior.* Cambridge, MA: Harvard University Press, 1937.

Merton, Thomas. *Contemplation in a World of Action.* Notre Dame, IN: University of Notre Dame Press, 1998.

Miller, Richard. *The iRest Program for Healing PTSD: A Proven-Effective Approach to Using Yoga Nidra Meditation and Deep Relaxation Techniques to Overcome Trauma.* Oakland, CA: New Harbinger Publications, 2015.

_____. *Yoga Nidra: A Meditative Practice for Deep Relaxation.* Boulder, CO: Sounds True, 2010.

Muller-Ortega, Paul Eduardo. *The Triadic Heart of Śiva: Kaula Tantricism of Abhinavagupta in the Non-Dual Shaivism of Kashmir.* Albany: State University of New York, 1988.

Ogden, Pat, Kekuni Minton, and Clare Pain. *Trauma and the Body: A Sensorimotor Approach to Psychotherapy.* New York: W.W. Norton, 2006.

Pierrakos, John. *Core Energetics: Developing the Capacity to Love and Heal.* Core Evolution Publishing, 2005.

Porges, Stephen W. *The Polyvagal Theory: Neurophysiological Foundations of Emotions, Attachment, Communication, and Self-Regulation.* New York: W.W. Norton, 2011.

Prendergast, John. *In Touch: How to Tune In to the Inner Guidance of Your Body and Trust Yourself.* Boulder, CO: Sounds True, 2015.

Ray, Reginald A. *Indestructible Truth.* Boston, MA: Shambhala, 2000.

_____. *Secret of the Vajra World: The Tantric Buddhism of Tibet.* Boston: Shambhala, 2001.

_____. *Touching Enlightenment: Finding Realization in the Body.* Boulder, CO: Sounds True, 2008.

Rosenberg, Jack, Marjorie Rand, and Diane Asay. *Body, Self, and Soul: Sustaining Integration.* Lake Worth, FL: Humanics Limited, 1985.

Rothschild, Babette. *The Body Remembers: The Psychophysiology of Trauma and Trauma Treatment.* New York: Norton, 2000.

_____. *The Body Remembers Casebook: Unifying Methods and Models in the Treatment of Trauma and PTSD.* New York: W.W. Norton, 2003.

Ryan, Regina Sara. *Only God.* Chino Valley, AZ: Hohm Press, 2015.

Scaer, Robert. *The Body Bears the Burden: Trauma, Dissociation, and Disease, Second Edition.* New York: Routledge, 2007.

Salmon, P. G., Saki E. Santorelli, and Jon Kabat-Zinn. "Intervention elements promoting adherence to mindfulness-based stress reduction programs in the clinical behavioral medicine setting." *Handbook of Health Behavior Change, Second Edition.* eds. Sally A. Shumaker, Eleanor B. Schron, Judith K. Ockene, and Wendy L. Bee. 239–268. New York: Springer, 1998.

Shaw, Miranda. *Passionate Enlightenment.* Princeton, NJ: Princeton University Press, 1994.

Siegel, Daniel J. *Mindsight: The New Science of Personal Transformation.* New York: Bantam Books, 2010.

_____. *Mind: A Journey to the Heart of Being Human.* New York: W.W. Norton, 2017.

_____. *The Mindful Brain: Reflection and Attunement in the Cultivation of Well-Being.* New York: W.W. Norton, 2007.

Simmer-Brown, Judith. *Dakini's Warm Breath: The Feminine Principle in Tibetan Buddhism.* Boston: Shambhala Publications, 2001.

Singleton, Mark. *Yoga Body: The Origins of Modern Posture Practice.* New York: Oxford University Press, 2010.

Sjoman, N. E. *The Yoga Tradition of the Mysore Palace, Second Edition.* New Delhi, India: Abhinav Publications, 1999.

Smith, Huston. *The World's Religions: Our Great Wisdom Traditions.* San Francisco: HarperSanFrancisco, 1991.

_____. *Why Religion Matters: The Fate of Human Spirit in an Age of Disbelief.* San Francisco: HarperSanFrancisco, 2001.

Solomon, Marion, and Daniel J. Siegel, eds. *Healing Trauma: Attachment, Mind, Body, and Brain.* W.W. Norton, 2003.

Sovatsky, Stuart. *Words from the Soul: Time, East/West Spirituality, and Psychotherapeutic Narrative.* Albany, NY: State University of New York Press, 1998.

Squire, Larry. *Fundamental Neuroscience, Fourth Edition.* Oxford, UK: Elsevier, 2013.

Svoboda, Robert. *Aghora: At the Left Hand of God.* Albuquerque, NM: Brotherhood of Life Inc., 1986.

_____. *Aghora II: Kundalini.* Albuquerque, NM: Brotherhood of Life Inc., 1993.

_____. *Aghora III: The Law of Karma.* Albuquerque, NM: Brotherhood of Life Inc., 1997.

Swami Muktibodhananda Saraswati, Swami Satyananda Saraswati, and Swami Svatmarama. *Hatha Yoga Pradipika.* Munger, Bihar, India: Yoga Publications Trust, 1998.

Swami Rama, Rudolph Ballentine, and Swami Ajaya. *Yoga and Psychotherapy: The Evolution of Consciousness.* Honesdale, PA: Himalayan Institute Press, 1976.

Thakar, Vimala. *On an Eternal Voyage.* Ahmedabad, India: Vimal Prakashan Trust, 1969.

Trungpa, Chögyam. *Cutting Through Spiritual Materialism*. Boston, MA: Shambhala, 1973.

van der Kolk, Bessel A. *The Body Keeps the Score: Brain, Mind, and Body in the Healing of Trauma*. New York: Penguin Books, 2014.

van der Kolk, Bessel A., Alexander C. McFarlane, and Lars Weiseith, eds. *Traumatic Stress: The Effects of Overwhelming Experience on Mind, Body, and Society*. New York: Guilford Press, 1996.

Vaughan-Lee, Llewellyn. *The Face Before I Was Born: A Spiritual Autobiography*. Inverness, CA: The Golden Sufi Center, 1997.

_____. *Awakening the World: A Global Dimension to Spiritual Practice*. Point Reyes, CA: The Golden Sufi Center, 2006.

Wallis, Christopher D., with Ekabhumi Ellik, illustrator. *Tantra Illuminated: The Philosophy, History, and Practice of a Timeless Tradition*. Petaluma, CA: Mattamayura Press, 2012.

Weintraub, Amy. *Yoga for Depression: A Compassionate Guide to Relieve Suffering through Yoga*. New York: Broadway Books, 2004.

_____. *Yoga Skills for Therapists: Effective Practices for Mood Management*. New York: W.W. Norton, 2012.

Welwood, John. *Awakening the Heart: East/West Approaches to Psychotherapy and the Healing Relationship*. Boston: Shambhala, 1983.

_____. *Perfect Love, Imperfect Relationships: Healing the Wound of the Heart*. Boston: Trumpeter, 2005.

_____. *Toward a Psychology of Awakening: Buddhism, Psychotherapy, and the Path of Personal and Spiritual Transformation*. Boston: Shambhala, 2002.

Woodman, Marion, and Elinor Dickson. *Dancing in the Flames: The Dark Goddess in the Transformation of Consciousness*. Boston: Shambhala, 1996.

STUDIES, RESEARCH, AND PERIODICALS

Abadi, M.S., et al. "Effect of Yoga on Children with Attention Deficit/ Hyperactivity Disorder." *Psychological Studies* 53, no. 2 (2008): 154–159.

Baer, Ruth A. "Mindfulness Training as a Clinical Intervention: A Conceptual and Empirical Review." *Clinical Psychology, Science and Review* 10 (June 2003): 125–143. doi: 10.1093/clipsy.bpg015.

Bangalore, N. Gangadhar, and Shivarama Varambally. "Yoga Therapy for Schizophrenia." *International Journal of Yoga* 5, no. 2 (2012): 85–91. doi: 10.4103/0973-6131.98212.

Barnes, P.M., et al. "Complementary and Alternative Medicine Use Among Adults and Children: United States, 2007." *CDC National Health Statistics Report* 12 (2008): Hyattsville, MD: National Center for Health Statistics, 2008. nccam.nih.gov/sites/nccam.nih.gov/files/news/nhsr12.pdf/

Berg, A. L., et al. "Patients' Perspective of Change Processes in Affect-Focused Body Psychotherapy for Generalized Anxiety Disorder." *Body, Movement, and Dance in Psychotherapy* 5, no. 2 (2010): 151–169.

Blanke, Olaf. "Multisensory Brain Mechanisms of Bodily Self-Consciousness." *Nature Reviews Neuroscience* 13, no. 8 (2012): 556–571. doi:10.1038/nrn3292.

Bonura, Kimberlee B., and David Pargman. "The Effects of Yoga Versus Exercise on Stress, Anxiety, and Depression in Older Adults." *International Journal of Yoga Therapy* 19, no. 1 (2009): 79–89. EBSCOhost.

Brewer, Judson A., et al. "Meditation Experience Is Associated with Differences in Default Mode Network Activity and Connectivity." *Proceedings of the National Academy of Sciences of the United States of America* 108, no. 50 (2011): 20254–20259. doi: 10.1073/pnas.1112029108.

Brisbon, Nicholas M., and Glenn A. Lowery. "Mindfulness and Levels of Stress: A Comparison of Beginner and Advanced Hatha Yoga Practitioners." *Journal of Religion and Health* 50, no. 4 (2011): 931–941. doi: 10.1007/s10943-009-9305-3.

Brown, Richard P., and Patricia L. Gerbarg. "Yoga Breathing, Meditation, and Longevity." *Annals of the New York Academy of Sciences* 1172 (2009): 54–62. doi: 10.1111/j.1749-6632.2009.04394.x.

Caplan, Mariana, Adriana Portillo, and Lynsie Seely. "Yoga Psychotherapy: The Integration of Western Psychological Theory and Ancient Yogic Wisdom." *The Journal of Transpersonal Psychology* 45, no. 2, (2013): 139–158.

Christopher, M. "A Broader View of Trauma: A Biopsychosocial-Evolutionary View of the Role of Traumatic Stress Response in the Emergence of Pathology and/or Growth." *Clinical Psychology Review* 24 (2004): 75–98. doi: 10.1016/j.cpr.2003.12.003 .

Cook, Alexandra, Joseph Spinazzola, et al. "Complex Trauma in Children and Adolescents," *Psychiatric Annals* 35, no. 5 (May 2005): 390–398. traumacenter.org/products/publications.php.

Dale, Lourdes P., et al. "Yoga Workshop Impacts Psychological Functioning and Mood of Women with Self-Reported History of Eating Disorders." *Eating Disorders: The Journal of Treatment & Prevention* 17, no.5 (2009): 422–434. doi: 10.1080/10640260903210222.

Damasio, Antonio R., et al. "The Somatic Marker Hypothesis and the Possible Functions of the Prefrontal Cortex." *Philosophical Transactions of the Royal Society of London B: Biological Sciences* 351, no. 1346 (October 29, 1996): 1413–1420. doi: 10.1098/rstb.1996.0125.

Davidson, Richard J., Jon Kabat-Zinn, et al. "Alterations in Brain and Immune Function Produced by Mindfulness Meditation." *Psychosomatic Medicine* 65, no. 4 (2003): 564–570. doi: 10.1097/01.PSY.0000077505.67574.E3.

Descilo, T., et. al. "Effects of a Yoga-Breath Intervention Alone and in Combination with an Exposure Therapy for Post-Traumatic Stress Disorder and Depression in Survivors of the 2004 Southeast Asia

Tsunami." *Acta Psychiatrica Scandinavica* 121, no. 4 (2010): 289–300. doi: 10.1111/j.1600-0447.2009.01466.x.

Diamond, Lisa M., et al. "Attachment Style, Vagal Tone, and Empathy During Mother-Adolescent Interactions." *Journal of Research on Adolescence* 22, no. 1 (2012): 165–184. doi: 10.1111/j.1532-7795.2011.00762.x.

Ditto, Blaine, Marie Eclache, and Natalie Goldman. "Short-Term Autonomic and Cardiovascular Effects of Mindfulness Body Scan Meditation." *Annals of Behavioral Medicine* 32, no. 3 (2006): 227–234. doi: 10.1207/s15324796abm3203_9.

Duraiswamy, G., et al. "Yoga Therapy as an Add-On Treatment in the Management of Patients with Schizophrenia: A Randomized Controlled Trial." *Acta Psychiatrica Scandinavica* 116, no. 3 (2007): 226–232. doi: 10.1111/j.1600-0447.2007.01032.x.

Eddy, Martha. "A Brief History of Somatic Practices and Dance: Historical Development of the Field of Somatic Education and Its Relationship to Dance." *Journal of Dance and Somatic Practices* 1, no. 1 (2009). doi: 10.1386/jdsp.1.1.5/1.

Emerson, David, et al. "Yoga Therapy in Practice: Trauma-Sensitive Yoga Principles, Practice, and Research." *International Journal of Yoga Therapy* 19 (2009): 123–128.

Epstein, Mark. "Meditative Transformations of Narcissism." *The Journal of Transpersonal Psychology* 18, no. 2 (1986): 143–158. atpweb.org/jtparchive/trps-18-86-02-143.pdf.

Farb, Norman A. S., et al. "Attending to the Present: Mindfulness Meditation Reveals Distinct Neural Modes of Self-Reference." *Social Cognitive and Affective Neuroscience* 2 (2007): 313–322. doi: 10.1093/scan/nsm030.

Ferrè, Elisa Raffaella, Christophe Lopez, and Patrick Haggard. "Anchoring the Self to the Body: Vestibular Contribution to the Sense of Self." *Psychological Science* 25, no. 11 (2014): 2106–2108. doi: 10.1177/0956797614547917.

Follette, Victoria M., et al. "Mindfulness and Trauma: Implications for Treatment." *Journal of Rational-Emotive and Cognitive-Behavior Therapy* 24, no. 1 (2006): 45–61. doi: 10.1007/s10942-006-0025-2.

Forbes, Bo, et al. "Using Integrative Yoga Therapeutics in the Treatment of Comorbid Anxiety and Depression." *International Journal of Yoga Therapy* 18, no. 1 (2008): 87–95. EBSCOhost.

Gallop, Ruth. "Failure of the Capacity for Self-Soothing in Women Who Have a History of Abuse and Self-Harm." *Journal of the American Psychiatric Nurses Association* 8, no. 1 (2002): 20–26. doi: 10.1067/mpn.2002.122425.

Gard, Tim, et al. "Effects of a Yoga-Based Intervention for Young Adults on Quality of Life and Perceived Stress: The Potential Mediating Roles of Mindfulness and Self-Compassion." *The Journal of Positive Psychology* 7, no. 3 (2012): 165–175. doi: 10.1080/17439760.2012.667144.

Gard, Tim, et al. "Potential Self-Regulatory Mechanisms of Yoga for Psychological Health." *Frontiers in Human Neuroscience* 8 (2014): 770. doi:10.3389/fnhum.2014.00770.

Gootjes, Liselotte., et al. "Cognitive Emotion Regulation in Yogic Meditative Practitioners: Sustained Modulation of Electrical Brain Potentials." *Journal of Psychophysiology* 25, no. 2 (2011): 87–94. doi: 10.1027/0269-8803/a000043.

Gotink, Rinske A., et al. "Mindfulness and Mood Stimulate Each Other in an Upward Spiral: A Mindful Walking Intervention Using Experience Sampling." *Mindfulness* 7, no. 5 (October 2016): 1114–1122.

Granath, Jens, et al. "Stress Management: A Randomized Study of Cognitive Behavioural Therapy and Yoga." *Cognitive Behaviour Therapy* 35, no. 1 (2006): 3–10. doi: 10.1080/16506070500401292.

Graziano, Michael. S., and Taylor W. Webb. "The Attention Schema Theory: A Mechanistic Account of Subjective Awareness." *Frontiers in Psychology* 6 (2015): 500. doi: 10.3389/fpsyg.2015.00500.

Harper, Jennifer. "Teaching Yoga in Urban Elementary Schools." *International Journal of Yoga Therapy* 20, no. 1 (2010): 99–109. EBSCOhost

Harrison, Linda J., et al. "Sahaja Yoga Meditation as a Family Treatment Programme for Children with Attention Deficit-Hyperactivity Disorder." *Clinical Child Psychology and Psychiatry* 9, no. 4 (2004): 479–497. doi: 10.1177/1359104504046155.

Hartelius, Glenn, Mariana Caplan, and Mary Anne Rardin. "Transpersonal Psychology: Defining the Past, Divining the Future." The Humanistic Psychologist 35, no. 2 (2007): 1–26.

Harvard Health Publications. "Yoga for Anxiety and Depression." *Harvard Mental Health Letter* Published April 2009, updated September 18, 2017. health.harvard.edu/mind-and-mood/yoga-for-anxiety-and-depression.

Hasenkamp, Wendy, and Lawrence W. Barsalou. "Effects of Meditation Experience on Functional Connectivity of Distributed Brain Networks." *Frontiers in Human Neuroscience* 6, no. 38 (2012). doi: 10.3389/fnhum.2012.00038.

Hasenkamp, Wendy, Christine D. Wilson-Mendenhall, Erica Duncan, and Lawrence W. Barsalou. "Mind Wandering and Attention During Focused Meditation: A Fine-Grained Temporal Analysis of Fluctuating Cognitive States." *NeuroImage* 59, no. 1 (2012): 750–760. doi: 10.1016/j.neuroimage.2011.07.008.

Hayano, Junichiro, et al. "Respiratory Sinus Arrhythmia: A Phenomenon Improving Pulmonary Gas Exchange and Circulatory Efficiency." *Circulation* 94, no. 4 (1996): 842–847. doi: 10.1161/01.cir.94.4.842.

Hölzel, Britta K. "Mindfulness Practice Leads to Increases in Regional Brain Grey-Matter Density." *Psychiatry Research* 191, no. 1 (2011): 36–43. doi: 10.1016/j.pscychresns.2010.08.006.

————. "Stress Reduction Correlates with Structural Changes in the Amygdala." *Social Cognitive and Affective Neuroscience* 5 (2010): 11–17. doi: 10.1093/scan/nsp034.

Hölzel, Britta K., et al. "How Does Mindfulness Meditation Work? Proposing Mechanisms of Action from a Conceptual and Neural Perspective." *Perspectives on Psychological Science* 6, no. 6 (2011): 537–559. doi: 10.1177/1745691611419671.

Impett, Emily A., Jennifer J. Daubenmier, and Allegra L. Hirschman. "Minding the Body: Yoga, Embodiment, and Well-Being." *Sexuality Research and Social Policy* 3, no. 4 (2006): 39–48. doi: 10.1525/srsp.2006.3.4.39.

Jensen, Pauline S., and Dianna T. Kenny. "The Effects of Yoga on the Attention and Behavior of Boys with Attention-Deficit/Hyperactivity Disorder (ADHD)." *Journal of Attention Disorders* 7, no. 4 (2004): 205–216. doi: 10.1177/108705470400700403.

Kinser, P.A., et al. "Feasibility, Acceptability, and Effects of Gentle Hatha Yoga for Women with Major Depression: Findings from a Randomized Controlled Mixed-Methods Study." *Archives of Psychiatric Nursing* 27, no. 3 (2013): 137–147. doi: 10.1016/j.apnu.2013.01.003.

Kirk, U., et al. "Mindfulness Training Increases Cooperative Decision Making in Economic Exchanges: Evidence from fMRI." *NeuroImage* 138 (2016): 274–283. doi: 10.1016/j.neuroimage.2016.05.075.

Koemeda-Lutz, Margit, et al. "Evaluation of the Effectiveness of Body Psychotherapy in Outpatient Settings (EEBP): A Multicenter Study in Germany and Switzerland." *Psychother. Psych. Med. Psychosom* 206, no. 56 (2006): 480–487. hakomiinstitute.com/Forum/Issue19-21/12EABPResearch.art2.pdf.

Koenig, Julian, et al. "Resting State Vagal Tone in Borderline Personality Disorder: A Meta-Analysis." *Progress in Neuro-Psychopharmacology and Biological Psychiatry* 64 (2016): 18–26. doi: 10.1016/j.pnpbp.2015.07.002.

Kok, Bethany E., et al. "How Positive Emotions Build Physical Health: Perceived Positive Social Connections Account for the Upward Spiral Between Positive Emotions and Vagal Tone." *Psychological Science* 24, no. 7 (2013): 1123–1132. doi: 10.1177/0956797612470827.

Lalande, Lloyd, et al. "Breathwork: An Additional Treatment Option for Depression and Anxiety." *Journal of Contemporary Psychotherapy* 42, no. 2 (2012): 113–119.

Lazar, Sara W., et al. "Functional Brain Mapping of the Relaxation Response and Meditation." *NeuroReport* 11, no. 7 (2000): 1581–1585. massgeneral.org/bhi/assets/pdfs/publications/lazar_2000_neuroreport.pdf.

Lazar, S. W., et al. "Meditation Experience Is Associated with Increased Cortical Thickness." *NeuroReport* 16, no. 17 (2005): 1893–1897.

Longaker, Kiranjit, and Gabriel Tornusciolo. "Yoga Group Therapy with Traumatized Adolescent Males." *International Journal of Yoga Therapy* 13 (2003): 75–82. EBSCOhost.

Lopez, Giovanni. "Why Verbal Psychotherapy Is Not Enough to Treat Post-Traumatic Stress Disorder: A Biosystemic Approach to Stress Debriefing."

Body, Movement, and Dance in Psychotherapy 6, no. 2 (2011): 129–143. doi: 10.1080/17432979.2011.583060.

Luders, Eileen., et al. "The Unique Brain Anatomy of Meditation Practitioners: Alterations in Cortical Gyrification." *Frontiers in Human Neuroscience* 6, no. 34 (2012): 1–9. doi: 10.3389/fnhum.2012.00034.

Masi, Christopher M., et al. "Respiratory Sinus Arrhythmia and Diseases of Aging: Obesity, Diabetes Mellitus, and Hypertension." *Biological Psychology* 74, no. 2 (2007): 212–223.

Mehling, Wolf E., et al. "Body Awareness: A Phenomenological Inquiry into the Common Ground of Mind-Body Therapies." *Philosophy, Ethics, and Humanities in Medicine* 6, no. 6 (2011). doi: 10.1186/1747-5341-6-6.

Miller, Richard C. "The Breath of Life: Through the Practice of Pranayama, the Regulation of the Breath, We Can Learn to Bring Forth and Direct the Spiritual Energy That Underlies All Life," *Yoga Journal* 116 (May/June 1994): 82. EBSCOhost.

Northoff, Georg, et al. "Self-Referential Processing in Our Brain: A Meta-Analysis of Imaging Studies on the Self." *NeuroImage* 31, no. 1 (2006): 440–457. doi: 10.1016/j.neuroimage.2005.12.002.

Ochsner, Kevin N., et al. "For Better or for Worse: Neural Systems Supporting the Cognitive Down-and-Up Regulation of Negative Emotion." *NeuroImage* 23 no. 2 (2004): 483–499. doi: 10.1016/j.neuroimage.2004.06.030.

Ochsner, Kevin N., and James J. Gross. "The Cognitive Control of Emotion." *Trends Cognitive Sciences* 9, no. 5 (2005): 242–249. doi: 10.1016/j.tics.2005.03.010.

Ogden, Pat, et al. "A Sensorimotor Approach to the Treatment of Trauma and Dissociation." *Psychiatric Clinics of North America* 29, no. 1 (2006): 263–279. doi: 10.1016/j.psc.2005.10.012.

Peng, Chung-Kang, et al. "Heart Rate Dynamics During Three Forms of Meditation." *International Journal of Cardiology* 95, no.1 (2004): 19–27. doi: 10.1016/j.ijcard.2003.02.006.

Philbin, Kait. "Transpersonal Integrative Yoga Therapy: A Protocol for Grief and Bereavement." *International Journal of Yoga Therapy* 19, no. 1 (2009): 129–141. EBSCOhost.

Pletikos, Mihovil, et al. "Temporal Specification and Bilaterality of Human Neocortical Topographic Gene Expression." *Neuron* 81, no. 2 (2014): 321–332. doi: 10.1016/j.neuron.2013.11.018.

Porges, Stephen W. "The Polyvagal Theory: Phylogenetic Substrates of a Social Nervous System." *International Journal of Psychophysiology* 42 (2001): 123–146.

Price, Cynthia. "Body-Oriented Therapy in Recovery from Child Sexual Abuse: An Efficacy Study." *Alternative Therapies in Health and Medicine* 11, no. 5 (2005): 46–57.

Price, Cynthia J., et al. "Mindful Awareness in Body-Oriented Therapy for Female Veterans with Post-Traumatic Stress Disorder Taking Prescription Analgesics for

Chronic Pain: A Feasibility Study." *Alternative Therapies in Health and Medicine* 13, no. 6 (2007): 32–40.

Pritchard, Mary, Patt Elison-Bowers, and Bobbie Birdsall. "Impact of Integrative Restoration (iRest) Meditation on Perceived Stress Levels in Multiple Sclerosis and Cancer Outpatients." *Stress and Health: Journal of the International Society for the Investigation of Stress* 26, no. 3 (2010): 233–237. doi: 10.1002/smi.1290.

Qin, Pengmin, and Georg Northoff. "How Is Our Self Related to Midline Regions and the Default-Mode Network?" *NeuroImage* 57, no. 3 (2011): 1221–1233. doi: 10.1016/j.neuroimage.2011.05.028.

Rozin, Paul, and Edward B. Royzman. "Negativity Bias, Negativity Dominance, and Contagion." *Personality and Social Psychology Review* 5, no. 4 (2001): 296–320. doi: 10.1207/s15327957pspr0504_2.

Sedlmeier, Peter., et al. "The Psychological Effects of Meditation: A Meta-Analysis." *Psychological Bulletin* 138, no. 6 (2012): 1139–1171. doi: 10.1037/a0028168.

Serber, Ellen. "Stress Management Through Yoga." *International Journal of Yoga Therapy* 10 (2000): 11–16. EBSCOhost.

Shapiro, David, and Karen Cline. "Mood Changes Associated with Iyengar Yoga Practices: A Pilot Study." *International Journal Of Yoga Therapy* 14, no. 1 (2004): 35–44. EBSCOhost.

Shelov, Danielle. V., et al. "A Pilot Study Measuring the Impact of Yoga on the Trait of Mindfulness." *Behavioural and Cognitive Psychotherapy* 37, no. 5 (2009): 595–598. doi: 10.1017/S1352465809990361.

Somel, Mehmet, et al. "Transcriptional Neoteny in the Human Brain." *Proceedings of the National Academy of Sciences* 106, no. 14 (2009): 5743–5748. doi: 10.1073/pnas.0900544106.

Sperduti, M., Pénélope Martinelli, and Pascale Piolino. "A Neurocognitive Model of Meditation Based on Activation Likelihood Estimation (ALE) Meta-Analysis." *Consciousness and Cognition* 21 (2012): 269–276. doi: 10.1016/j.concog.2011.09.019.

Spinazzola, Joseph, et al. "Application of Yoga in Residential Treatment of Traumatized Youth." *Journal of the American Psychiatric Nurses Association* 17, no. 6 (2011): 431–444. doi: 10.1177/1078390311418359.

Steckler, Laura, and Courtenay Young. "Depression and Body Psychotherapy." *International Journal of Psychotherapy* 13, no. 2 (2009): 32–41. courtenay-young.co.uk/courtenay/articles/Steckler_Young_Depression_BP.pdf.

Streeter, Chris C., et al. "Effects of Yoga Versus Walking on Mood, Anxiety, and Brain GABA Levels: A Randomized Controlled MRS Study." *The Journal of Alternative and Complementary Medicine* 16, no. 11 (2010): 1145–1152. doi: 10.1089/acm.2010.0007.

Swart, A. "Partner Yoga for Establishing Boundaries in Relationship: A Transpersonal Somatic Approach." *International Journal of Yoga Therapy* 21 (2011): 123–128. EBSCOhost.

Tang, Yi-Yuan, Britta Hölzel, and Michael Posner. "The Neuroscience of Mindfulness Meditation." *Nature Reviews Neuroscience* 16, no. 4 (2015): 213–225. doi: 10.1038/nrn3916.

Telles, Shirley. "Yoga Reduces Symptoms of Distress in Tsunami Survivors in the Andaman Islands." *Evidence-Based Complementary & Alternative Medicine* 4, no. 4 (2007): 503–509. doi: 10.1093/ecam/nem069.

Telles, Shirley, et al. "Post-Traumatic Stress Symptoms and Heart Rate Variability in Bihar Flood Survivors Following Yoga: A Randomized Controlled Study." *BMC Psychiatry* 10, no. 18 (2010): 1–10. doi: 10.1186/1471-244X-10-18.

van der Kolk, Bessel A. "Clinical Implications of Neuroscience Research in PTSD." *Annals of the New York Academy of Sciences* 1071 (July 26, 2006): 277–293. traumacenter.org/products/publications.php.

van der Kolk, Bessel A. "Post-Traumatic Therapy in the Age of Neuroscience." *Psychoanalytic Dialogues* 12, no. 3 (2002): 381. doi: 10.1080/10481881209348674

van der Kolk, Bessel A. "The Assessment and Treatment of Complex PTSD." In *Traumatic Stress*, ed. Rachel Yehuda. Arlington, VA: American Psychiatric Press, 2002.

van der Kolk, Bessel A. "The Body Keeps Score: Memory and the Evolving Psychobiology of Post-Traumatic Stress." *Harvard Review of Psychiatry* 1, no. 5 (1994): 253–265. traumacenter.org/products/publications.php.

Vestergaard-Poulsen, Peter, et al. "Long-Term Meditation Is Associated with Increased Gray Matter Density in the Brain Stem." *NeuroReport* 20, no. 2 (2009): 170–174. doi: 10.1097/WNR.0b013e328320012a.

Visceglia, Elizabeth, and Stephen Lewis. "Yoga Therapy as an Adjunctive Treatment for Schizophrenia: A Randomized, Controlled Pilot Study." *The Journal of Alternative and Complementary Medicine* 17, no. 7 (2011). 601–607. doi: 10.1089/acm.2010.0075.

Walsh, Roger. "The Search for Synthesis." *Journal of Humanistic Psychology* 32, no. 1 (1992): 19–45.

Wimmer, G. Elliott, and Daphna Shohamy. "Preference by Association: How Memory Mechanisms in the Hippocampus Bias Decisions." *Science* 338, no. 6104 (2012): 270–273. doi: 10.1126/science.1223252.

Wolever, R.Q., et al. "Effective and Viable Mind-Body Stress Reduction in the Workplace: A Randomized Controlled Trial." *Journal and Occupational Health Psychology* 17, no. 2 (2012): 246–258. doi: 10.1037/a0027278.

Xie, Xiyao, et al. "How Do You Make Me Feel Better? Social Cognitive Emotion Regulation and the Default Mode Network," *NeuroImage* 134 (July, 2016): 270–280. doi: 10.1016/j.neuroimage.2016.04.015.

"2016 Yoga in America Study Conducted by *Yoga Journal* and Yoga Alliance." Yoga Alliance website. Published January 13, 2016. yogaalliance. org/2016yogainamericastudy.

INDEX